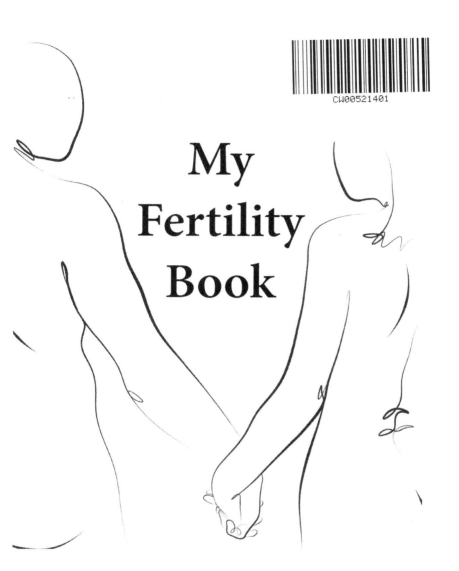

My Fertility Book

SHEILA LAMB
Founder of My Fertility Specialist magazine

Reviews

A comprehensive guide to often baffling, and sometimes upsetting, infertility terminology and jargon. I always tell my clients they're going to have to get up to speed fast and this book will be hugely helpful and comforting in explaining complex terminology in plain English. I thoroughly recommend it.

Dee Armstrong, Fertility Coach & Counsellor, The Natural Fertility Centre, Edinburgh, Scotland

Stunningly comprehensive. I wish I'd had this impressive guide 16 years ago. I would have soaked it up, because any practical research felt as if I had some control over the IVF process. While highly assured, it also embraces nice touches of humour e.g. sperm affected by alcohol don't swim in a straight line! I found terms for new treatments that didn't exist for me back then, such as Endometrial Scratch. I was also moved to learn that my daughter was a Rainbow Baby - born after miscarriage.

Diane Chandler, author of 'Moondance' and 'The Road to Donestsk: How hard can it be to do good?

Whether you are trying to conceive naturally or embarking on IVF, this book is your 'must have' resource. Once you start your fertility journey, you are suddenly thrown into a world that can be utterly terrifying, full of terminology that on the face of it looks like a foreign language. A fertility journey is hard enough without feeling confused and alienated when confronted with the utterly dumfounding words routinely used in forums, by your doctor and by your specialist. This gem of a book puts you firmly back in control and allows you to navigate your fertility journey with confidence. I will be 'prescribing' this fabulous resource as a 'trying to conceive companion' for ALL of my patients.

Kate Davies – Fertility Nurse Consultant & Coach (RGN,Bsc (Hons), FP Cert) Your Fertility Journey

As a fertility reflexologist there is never enough time to browse the internet to be able to understand all the fertility jargon. This book is amazing, wonderful and a great valuable reference which will stay forever in my practice bookshelf in use! This book is easy to refer on the day to day when my clients have specific questions which I'm not always able to answer. I highly recommend this book for anyone who is going through this tiring and emotional journey of becoming a parent, or anyone supporting couples on their journey to parenthood.

Cécile M. Rainsford -MAR @ Ped à Terre Reflexology

My Fertility Book is a fabulous resource to have if you are interested in, or involved in, the world of Fertility. Sheila Lamb includes numerous useful and clear definitions and descriptions of terms and lingo used in the Fertility world. I often tell my clients who embark on a journey of family creation, that it will feel as if you need to learn a new language. Ms. Lamb's book is a tool I can offer to my clients, in order to help their learning curve be less overwhelming. Thanks to Ms. Lamb for a highly important and useful book in the complex world of assisted reproduction.

Cheryl Lister - Fertility Journey Coach, Private Practice

This book is going to help so, so many women and couples in general. It is written in a way that everybody can understand and feel a bit more in control and comfortable throughout their fertility journey. I have been a midwife for over 10 years and mostly working with women with fertility problems or treatments during pregnancy/high risk pregnancy. Despite my degree and experience as a midwife and a KG hypnobirthing teacher I have had times where I found difficulties explaining concepts or techniques to my patients in a way they can understand. But, also from my personal experience going through some fertility issues myself, I wish I had this book to hand! This book will make a huge difference and positive impact on any couple going through the hard and heart-breaking journey of infertility.

Paula Lavandeira - RGM Founder of The Nurtured Munchkin

My Fertility Book

All the fertility and infertility
explanations you will ever need,
from A to Z

Sheila Lamb

Published in 2018 by MFSBooks.com

ISBN: 978-1-9993035-1-8

A CIP catalogue record for this book is available from the British Library.

About the Author

Hi, I am the author Sheila Lamb and, for over six years, I was on a journey very similar to the one you're quite possibly on right now. Dealing with fertility issues is not easy emotionally, and it is made much harder because you have to become a medical expert overnight. I was fortunate that I had a background as a nurse and midwife, but even I struggled to understand the language frequently used by fertility doctors and nurses, and what people were writing about in online forums. Just what do AFC, LPD and PUPO stand for? And what is azoospermia, ovarian reserve and sonohysterogram? After our third ICSI cycle (that's intracytoplasmic sperm injection) was successful, nine anxiety ridden months later, we welcomed our miracle daughter into our lives.

Infertility is a life-changing event and I never forgot our battle and wanted to help others in some way, so I combined my two passions – writing and fertility – and founded an online magazine called My Fertility Specialist, with the help of many amazing fertility experts and fabulous women who kindly shared their stories. Although the magazine helped many people, I wanted to concentrate more on supporting just one area of the infertility battle, and one area that seemed to cause massive anxiety and frustration was understanding medical terms, investigations and fertility treatments. During medical appointments, the doctor or nurse provides so much information that it is impossible to take everything in and be confident enough to ask questions that will help your understanding. It's only afterwards that you realise you can't remember anything that was said. This is why I've written My Fertility Book; an in-depth glossary of all the information you need, clearly explained and in one easily accessible place.

Wherever you are on your journey, I hope you find this book useful and I truly hope that you realise your dream of becoming a parent, however it happens for you.

Dedicated to our darling miracle daughter,
Jessica
-x-

Contents

Acknowledgements

I'm not sure where the line is drawn as to who should be acknowledged in a book such as this, so I'm going to acknowledge every single person who has encouraged, supported, showed an interest and listened to me, as well as all those who have contributed in one way or another. So here goes…..

From my personal life, the first person I would like to thank is my husband who has always said I should write a book about our fertility experience; I'm not sure he expected it to take as long as it has, but he has been patient and as he is great at all the technical stuff, I really do owe him a lot for helping me, so thank you very much. Equal joint first place is our daughter Jessica, who regularly put up with me putting various Disney movies on again and again… so I could grab a couple of hours of writing time, but who frequently asked "How is your book coming on Mummy?" My parents, John and Freda, who helped immensely during our fertility struggles and who have known since I was a little girl that I wanted to be a writer. My sisters Angela and Judy who encouraged me to finish this book. My friends who asked politely how the book was coming on and then, to their credit, looked interested when I told them the latest update and encouraged me to keep going: thank you so much to Michelle Starkey, Claudia Sievers, Angie Conlon, Diane Bell, Maria Bagao, Heidi Fitch, Kat Konieczny, Shelley Treen, Caroline Thyer-Jones. Linda Sheppard, Melissa Werry, Emily Austin, Katharine Moore, Lisa Bond, Sue Monaghan, Gill Robinson and Jackie Chidwick.

My fertility family have to be the most supportive, caring, kind group of people I have ever come across. I met so many wonderful women and men when I was putting together my online magazine and, when I took a year out and then got back in contact with them when I was writing the book, they welcomed me back with open arms and it felt like I had never been away. So very special thanks to: Dr Mahadeo Bhide, MD, MRCOG who kindly reviewed and gave me his expert feedback on some of the terms in the book, and made many helpful suggestions during our often very late-night chats, Anya Sizer from Fertility Network UK and author of 'Fertile Thinking', Jessica Hepburn, founder of Fertility Fest and author of 'The Pursuit of Motherhood' and '21 Miles', Stephanie Roth from Your fertile self, Kate Davies from Your fertility journey, Nicola Salmon feminist fertility coach & acupuncturist and author of 'Nurture Fertility Journal', Helena Tubridy fertility coach & hypnotherapist, Sarah Holland from Fertile Mindset, Angela Heap from Fertile Ground Nutrition, Lisa Attfield from Fertility Yoga, Diane Chandler author of 'Moondance' and 'The Road to Donetsk', Emma Cannon acupuncturist and author of a number of books including 'The Baby Making Bible', Gordana Petrovic from Acumedicare, Clare Spink from Fertility Massage, Rachel Campbell from Sprout and Co, Bianca Smith from Where's my stork? and author of 'IVF: a detailed guide' and 'My Ukrainian Surrogacy Journey,' Yemisi Adegbile from Concept Fertility clinic, Natalie Silverman from Fertility Podcast, Tracey Sainsbury from The London Women's clinic and co-author of 'Making friends with your fertility', Kristen Darcy coach and speaker and author of a number of books including 'Girlfriend to Girlfriend: a fertility companion' and Dee Armstrong from The Natural Fertility Centre.

Since starting to write the book, my fertility family has widened further and the encouragement and interest from these wonderful fertility experts has been amazing. Huge thanks to: Dr Emma Brodzinski therapist and fertility coach, Finola Mcconville from Loving Touch Therapies, Aileen Feeney CEO Fertility Network UK, Toni Weschler from Taking Charge of Your Fertility and Fertility author of the book of the same name, Zita West from Zita West Fertility Clinic and author of many books, including 'Guide to fertility and assisted conception' and Dany Griffiths Freedom Fertility Coach.

I also have to thank Phillip Reed, who came to my rescue when the first illustrator I found let me down. I do believe that things happen for a reason though, and although at the time I was panic stricken and didn't know how I would find another illustrator, along came Phillip who is a member of an indie author Facebook group I'm also part of. His wonderfully artistic, easy-on-the-eye illustrations help to explain some of the medical terms, whilst his cartoons will, I'm sure, bring a smile to your face. This is a little bit about Phillip:

After failing to impress girls at high school with drawings of cute cartoon animals, Phillip put aside his dreams of being an artist and took on what his mother described as 'a proper job'. He then spent the next thirty years working in various administrative and management positions, but was never able to repress the creative impulse. Feeling unfulfilled, he gained qualifications in art and creative writing. After cautiously drip-feeding his artwork to work colleagues for many years, he finally succumbed to their constant taunts of 'you're wasted here!' and decided that maybe his career did lie elsewhere. Phillip has since been published in magazines and has written and illustrated children's books. He lives in the small Essex village of Mistley, overlooking the River Stour and spends his spare time with his two greatest loves; his children and his irrepressible imagination.

To contact Phillip, email info@philliplreed.com

Foreword

Sheila Lamb has written this must-read book for anyone thinking about starting a family, who is currently going through infertility struggles or is supporting people on their journey. Anyone that has experienced this, will know just how many confusing terms and abbreviations are used. Sheila has explained so many fertility terms in simple and jargon free language, which will without doubt, save the reader much frustration and many hours trawling the internet searching for information. In addition to all the explanations, Sheila has included some wonderful illustrations to further help explain medical terms, such as egg collection, donor insemination, and intracytoplasmic sperm injection (ICSI). I particularly like the cartoon of an embryologist.

I like that Sheila has steered clear of giving advice or making any suggestions as to what people should do regards treatment. As we are well aware, no two people are the same and treatment should be personalised, so readers must ensure they seek the advice of their medical practitioner about their own personal situation. That said, the book contains a wealth of information and does provide the reader with some different viewpoints to consider regarding the benefits of some treatments, particularly where the evidence on their effect are inconclusive as to whether they provide benefit or not.

Although this book is a comprehensive glossary of terms, Sheila has also shared some of her own personal experiences of infertility, such as dealing with a miscarriage, the two week wait and the emotional impact of fertility treatment. I am sure this will be extremely helpful to the reader, whether you are a woman, man or supporting someone through their journey.

Lastly, as the CEO of Fertility Network UK, I am delighted that Sheila has offered to make a donation from every book sold in the UK. As a charity we rely on donations; through buying this book, you are helping us to help more people who are experiencing fertility problems. So, I would like to thank you very much.

Aileen Feeney, CEO Fertility Network UK

Introduction

If you are reading this book then the chances are that either you or you and your partner together are looking for information to help make your own family. Or you may be supporting someone either professionally as a coach or counsellor, or personally – a friend – who is finding it challenging to start a family. Families are made in many different ways; some need a little bit of medical intervention whilst others need more than two people to provide the ingredients. When we were children I bet none of us thought that we would need any help to have a baby; you never intended to be in this position and it definitely isn't your fault. It isn't anyone's fault. One of the hardest things about having fertility problems is that unlike with many diseases (infertility is recognised by the World Health Organisation or WHO), there is no one cause. Unlike any other disease, the reason for it can be down to two people, further complicating matters.

Another complication with the whole area of fertility that leads to frustration on our part is that very often there are at least two camps of belief (sometimes three), in the medical profession – believers, non-believers and then the maybes. For example, some doctors believe that natural killer cells are associated with miscarriages and others say there is no connection at all. There often aren't studies to prove or disprove treatments and this is why it is so frustrating for those looking for answers.

I'm afraid I don't have all the answers; but I am someone who has been through my own fertility battle, and this is important when helping others and knowing what is needed. With my medical knowledge and own personal experience, I have explained the terms using straightforward, 'plain English'. I use the analogy that this book is like a recipe book – you dip in and out of a recipe book as you need to and cook the recipes you like the sound

21

of. Similarly, you probably won't need to know every term in this book and you probably won't read it from cover to cover (but you can if you want to); simply read the terms you want to find out about then dip into it when you come across a new term, or your journey takes you down a new path and you want to find out new information. Please be sure to read 'The miracle of mother nature' a few pages, on as this explains very well why it is a miracle that any woman gets pregnant in the first place.

One thing I have been very careful not to do is to give my opinion because this wouldn't be fair or right. I have, however, sometimes passed on my thoughts and experiences from my journey, things that made us laugh and cry and things I learnt, because I found this sort of 'advice' very helpful and helped me feel less alone. These parts you will find in a text box labelled 'Sheila says'.

I hope you like the illustrations as much as I do – I really wanted them to bring something extra to the book but I didn't want them to offend anyone, because everything to do with fertility is very personal and quite embarrassing. I also wanted to try and lighten the tone of the book – a book on fertility medical and non-medical terms doesn't really sound that exciting, does it? So, I couldn't help but include some cartoons and I hope they give you a laugh or two. Please note: the illustrations are not to scale as such, they are an artist's impression only. I also hope you find the fertility facts on the alphabet letter pages interesting.

When I was putting this book together I wrote it as if you and I were sitting down together chatting about the fertility terms. I also assumed it would mainly be women reading this book because we are generally the ones who do the reading and research – hence I wrote it to 'you/your' and not to 'woman/women'.

Knowing how stressful everything is when it's not straightforward to make a baby, it's very important to me that you can pick up this book as and when you need it and understand the explanation immediately. All the terms in this book are relevant regardless of where you live in the world – fertility issues and treatment are the same whether you come from Australia or Zanzibar. Because I live in the UK the spelling and grammar are in UK English, but I have tried as far as possible to include the US spelling of key words so I hope you will understand one or the other.

I have to say, some terms caused me much angst, e.g.: 'Is this to do with fertility or not? It mentions being "pregnant" but also "difficult to get pregnant".' Therefore, I have made what I hope is the right decision and included the term, because this book is for you, not for me, and I didn't feel it was my place not to give you the option of knowing this particular piece of information. I humbly apologise if any of these terms cause you upset and I hope you will forgive me. Also, I don't want this book to endorse or advertise any products. However, brand name products are mentioned on forums and in support groups so I have included the common ones and explained what they are. I emphasise again that I am not endorsing these products and have nothing to do with the companies. If you want to find out more about the product, please visit the company's website.

I think every country has a charity working on behalf of those who find themselves battling with infertility, and they do an absolutely amazing job and obviously rely heavily on donations. In the UK, Fertility Network UK is the charity and I am delighted to tell you that for every copy of this book sold in the UK, a donation will be made to Fertility Network UK.

Lastly, I appreciate that advances are being made all the time and more is being understood every day about infertility and fertility (thankfully), so this book will be updated in the future. If you would like to be kept right up to date with fertility news as it happens, please sign up to my newsletter by visiting www.mfsbooks.com

How to get the most out of this book

The first thing to say is this book definitely does not replace seeking the advice of healthcare professionals.

As it's a glossary of medical and non-medical terms with easy-to-understand explanations, it is presented in alphabetical order. The term is listed first, followed by its abbreviations or acronym if it has one. An acronym is an abbreviation formed from the initial letters of other words and pronounced as a word, and they're widely used in medicine. Often a term is called a number of different things and where this happens I have included a reference to go to that other term to find out more information; if I had repeated everything the book would have been twice as long as it is.

You may like to use this book with my free ebook called 'The Best Fertility Jargon Buster; the most concise A-Z list of fertility abbreviations and acronyms you will ever need', because the jargon buster book lists the abbreviation/acronym first followed by the full name of the term meaning, making it easy to find what you're looking for.

As already mentioned, in the explanations I have used 'you' and 'your' rather than 'woman' or 'female', as I anticipate it will more likely be women who read and use this book than men (apologies to those men who are reading it).

For the sake of avoiding repetition and boring you, there are a few very common fertility terms that are mentioned many hundreds of times in this book, so I have often used their abbreviation rather than the whole word, but a full explanation is still given in the book. They are:

Assisted reproductive technology – abbreviated to ART

In vitro fertilisation – abbreviated to IVF

Intrauterine insemination – abbreviated to IUI

Intracytoplasmic injection – abbreviated to ICSI

Ovarian Hyperstimulation Syndrome - abbreviated to OHSS

Polycystic ovarian/ovary Syndrome - abbreviated to PCOS

Uterus/womb are the same organ

Lastly, if you find this book helpful, please tell others who you know or you come across so that you have also helped them, and if you would like to reach more people, please leave a book review on the bookstore you purchased it from. Thank you.

The miracle of Mother Nature

How two tiny cells, an egg and a sperm, actually make a baby is nothing short of miraculous. When we decide we would like to start a family, we assume that after having sex at about the right time of the month, a couple of million sperm will dash off all eager to find the one egg that has quite recently popped out of our ovary. One eager sperm will win the race, fertilise the egg and the baby-to-be will snuggle down into your womb for nine months. But that's not the whole story! To make a baby involves so many ingredients in the correct quantity being added to the mix at the right time and in the right order – if anything isn't absolutely spot on, it's impossible for the egg and sperm to create your baby. Below is the sequence of events that has to happen and, when you get to the end, I'm sure you'll agree that every one of us is an absolute miracle.

- The hormone in your brain (GnRH) and the hormones (FSH and LH) in your pituitary gland must all be made and released in the right quantity to start follicle and egg development in your ovary

- The hormone in the man's brain (GnRH) and the hormones (FSH and LH) in his pituitary gland must all be made and released in the right quantity to make the hormone testosterone in his testicles

- There must be the correct level of testosterone in order to start making sperm in his testicles

- The temperature in his testicles and scrotum must be correct in order to make sperm and for sperm to mature

- The egg in your dominant follicle must have the correct number of chromosomes (23) and everything else must be normal

- Sperm must have the correct number of chromosomes (23) and everything must be normal
- The hormones made in your pituitary gland and in your ovary (oestrogen/estrogen) must be able to mature the egg
- Under the influence of oestrogen/estrogen, your womb lining must be thickening adequately
- The level of oestrogen/estrogen must be correct to bring about the surge of LH that will finally mature the egg
- 28 to 36 hours after this surge, the egg must pop out of the follicle – this is ovulation
- The follicle becomes the corpus luteum which continues to make oestrogen/estrogen but now also makes enough of the hormone progesterone to prepare your womb lining for implantation
- The minute hair-like structures (cilia) must be able to waft the egg from your ovary into the opening of your Fallopian tube
- Your Fallopian tube must be clear and not blocked
- Sperm must be able to physically move from where they are made in his testicles to the epididymis, where they mature, and into the vas deferens then the urethra, where ejaculation takes place
- There must be nothing to block the sperm's way
- Sperm must be able to swim vigorously in a straight line from your vagina, through your cervix and cervical mucus, through your womb and up into your Fallopian tube to meet the egg
- The egg must give off chemical signals to guide the sperm
- Sperm must be able to get through the cells that surround

your egg and bind with the shell, or zona pellucida, of the egg

- One sperm must then be able to react to certain chemicals and release its DNA with its 23 chromosomes into your egg – this is fertilisation

- The egg changes its outer membrane so that no other sperm can get in

- The fertilised egg, or zygote, must be able to divide first into two cells

- As it begins its three to four-day journey down your Fallopian tube to your womb, the zygote must continue to divide into four cells, then eight cells and when it is 16 cells, it is technically called a 'morula'

- When it is a bundle of cells with a small cavity between them it is called a 'blastocyst'. On reaching your womb roughly five days after fertilisation, the blastocyst hatches from its shell

- Providing your womb lining is receptive and has developed properly, the hatched blastocyst must implant itself into your womb lining – it is now an embryo

- The embryo must continue to develop properly so that part of its cells become the placenta and the other cells make your baby.

Female reproductive organs and the glands that make her fertility hormones (this is not to scale and is purely an artistic impression)

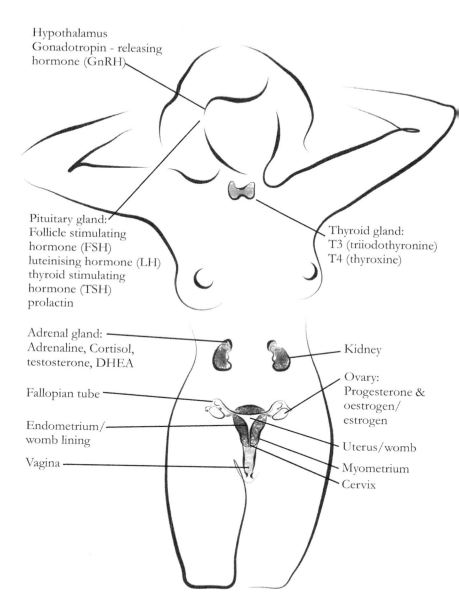

Hypothalamus
Gonadotropin - releasing
hormone (GnRH)

Pituitary gland:
Follicle stimulating
hormone (FSH)
luteinising hormone (LH)
thyroid stimulating
hormone (TSH)
prolactin

Thyroid gland:
T3 (triiodothyronine)
T4 (thyroxine)

Adrenal gland:
Adrenaline, Cortisol,
testosterone, DHEA

Kidney

Fallopian tube

Ovary:
Progesterone &
oestrogen/
estrogen

Endometrium/
womb lining

Uterus/womb

Vagina

Myometrium

Cervix

Male reproductive organs and the glands that make his fertility hormones (this is not to scale and is purely an artistic impression)

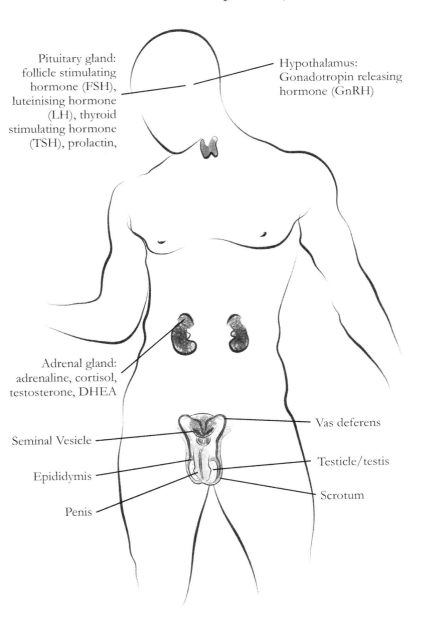

Pituitary gland: follicle stimulating hormone (FSH), luteinising hormone (LH), thyroid stimulating hormone (TSH), prolactin,

Hypothalamus: Gonadotropin releasing hormone (GnRH)

Adrenal gland: adrenaline, cortisol, testosterone, DHEA

Seminal Vesicle

Epididymis

Penis

Vas deferens

Testicle/testis

Scrotum

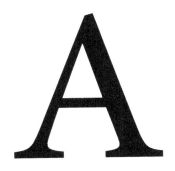

ACUPUNCTURE

to

AZOOSPERMIA

The WHO has stated: 'Infertility in women was ranked the 5th highest serious global disability (among populations under the age of 60).'

Acupuncture

Acupuncture is an ancient Chinese medicine treatment. Traditional practitioners believe that the body can be mapped with energy channels called meridians. Fine needles are inserted at points around your body to correct imbalances in energy or 'qi', which flows around the body in meridians. The opinions and findings as to how acupuncture helps fertility are inconclusive. Those who believe say acupuncture can help with:

• regulating your menstrual cycle

• improving blood circulation to your womb and ovaries

• aiding embryo implantation

• reducing stress

• regulating hormones.

For the men, it is believed it can improve sperm count and motility (see 'Semen Analysis'). See also 'Electro Stim Acupuncture'.

Adenomyosis

This disease occurs when endometrial tissue, which normally lines your uterus, exists within and grows into the muscular wall. It continues to act in the same way – thickening, breaking down and bleeding – during each menstrual cycle. It can cause an enlarged uterus and painful, heavy periods. Often you will also have endometriosis and it is believed that adenomyosis may contribute towards infertility. See 'Endometriosis' for more information.

Adhesions

Sometimes called scar tissue, adhesions are bands of tissue that stick tissue and organs together. Anything that leads to an inflammatory response, such as surgery, endometriosis or infection, can cause adhesions. Adhesions inside or around the Fallopian tubes, uterus and ovaries are likely to lead to infertility or an ectopic pregnancy.

The below is not to scale and is an artistic impression of your reproductive system.

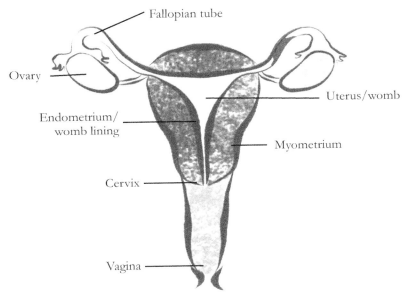

Adrenal Glands/Adrenaline

The adrenal glands are located on top of your kidneys and release certain hormones in response to stress, namely adrenaline and cortisol. The adrenals also release androgen hormones relevant to fertility: DHEA (dehydroepiandrosterone), testosterone and androstenedione. The adrenal glands also influence hormones from other parts of your body.

If you, and your partner, live in a constant stressful state, this causes overworked adrenals, which results in high levels of adrenaline and cortisol, which in turn affects the hormone progesterone, essential for getting pregnant. Adrenaline also causes the pituitary gland to release higher levels of prolactin, which may contribute to infertility.

Advanced Maternal Age – AMA

The formal medical threshold (which many of us find surprising) is over 35 years of age.

Alcohol

It has been said for many years that alcohol affects the fertility of men and women but we all know women who do get pregnant without any problems who, in their younger days, spent most weekends recovering from a hangover. But if you are trying to get pregnant or planning on trying within the next few months, it would be advisable not only for you, but for your future child, if you either cut down or had a complete break. This is the same for your partner. For you, drinking more than five glasses of alcohol a week may cause the following:

- amenorrhea – see 'Amenorrhea' for further information
- dysmenorrhea (painful periods)
- irregular periods.

For men, excessive alcohol makes their sperm act as if they are also drunk in that they don't swim in a straight line. I'm being serious! As sperm are made constantly, if a man gives up the alcohol or cuts down, the newly produced sperm will swim in a straight line. Alcohol can also have the following effects:

- lowers testosterone levels
- affects sperm quality and quantity
- reduces libido and causes impotence.

Amenorrhea – Primary and Secondary

Primary amenorrhea is when you have not started menstruating by the age of 14 and have no secondary sexual characteristics, such as breasts, pubic hair etc, or no menstruation by the age of 16 regardless of secondary sexual characteristics. It is uncommon and the cause is usually due to an underlying developmental issue. If you have primary amenorrhea you should be referred to a reproductive endocrinologist.

Secondary amenorrhea is where there has been no menstruation for the total of at least three previous menstrual cycle lengths, or at least six months if you have previously had a menstrual cycle, and if you are between puberty and the menopause. This is more common than primary and is usually due to imbalances in the endocrine system, specifically the hormones necessary for reproduction. This may also occur after major weight loss through rapid dieting, anorexia nervosa etc.

American Society for Reproductive Medicine – ASRM

This is a group of fertility experts who want to advance the 'art, science and practise' of reproductive medicine. Although it was started in America, the members now come from around the world. They have an annual meeting as well as courses, workshops, seminars and publications. The European equivalent is ESHRE (European Society of Human Reproduction and Embryology).

Andrologist

This is a doctor who has trained as a urologist and then gone on to specialise in the treatment of conditions affecting male fertility, such as low or absent sperm count.

The below is not to scale and is an artistic impression of the male reproductive system.

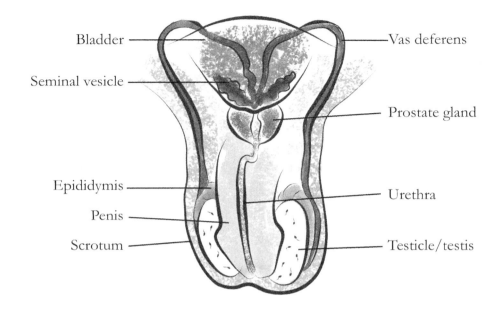

Anejaculation

This is when a man is unable to ejaculate semen. It may occur only in certain situations or all the time. It is due to the prostate gland and seminal ducts not being able to release semen. Possible causes include:

- injury to the pelvis or spinal column
- diabetes
- prostate surgery for cancer
- multiple sclerosis
- psychological factors such as stress, anxiety and relationship issues.

Angel Baby

A baby who has been lost during a pregnancy and is now a little angel in heaven. Some people go as far as to see them as their guardian angels who are alive, well and happy.

Anovulation – AO

This is when your ovaries do not release an egg (oocyte) during a menstrual cycle so ovulation does not occur. It may cause menstrual cycles to be irregular or for you to have no periods at all. It can be caused by conditions that affect the following glands: thyroid, adrenal, hypothalamus and pituitary. All these glands are relevant in controlling the hormonal balance that leads to ovulation. Other causes include:

- polycystic ovarian syndrome (PCOS)
- being overweight or underweight
- excessive exercise
- high levels of stress
- premature menopause, also called 'premature ovarian failure' or POF.

Because there are a number of causes, treatment will vary and will be aimed at treating the underlying cause. It is important you see a specialist to get an accurate diagnosis.

Anti-cardiolipin Antibodies – ACA

Cardiolipin is a molecule (a group of two or more atoms bonded together) which is present in your blood platelets (platelets help your blood to clot if you cut yourself) and other cell membranes. In some people, their body sees cardiolipin as a foreign body so they automatically produce anti-cardiolipin antibodies or ACAs to fight and destroy cardiolipin. You may have these ACAs but don't know this because you don't have any symptoms and this is probably because the levels are quite low. However, if you have high levels of ACAs, you may have symptoms such as:

- unexplained infertility
- unexplained miscarriages
- unexplained stillbirths
- blood clots.

People who have an autoimmune disease such as Systemic Lupus Erythematosus (SLE) or anti-phospholipid syndrome will show high levels of ACAs.

When you start having fertility tests done because you can't get pregnant, your doctor may discuss you having a blood test to see what your levels are. The test may need to be repeated if it comes back as borderline because minor illnesses, such as a cold or flu, can affect the level of antibodies. If your levels are high, your doctor will advise the most appropriate treatments to help control the number of ACAs in your blood and reduce the risk of you having blood clots such as deep vein thrombosis (DVT). Such medication could be baby aspirin, heparin or Clexane injections; prednisone/prednisolone is an anti-inflammatory and cyclosporin stops the antibodies.

Antidepressants

These drugs may affect your fertility by causing irregular periods, interfering with the hormones concerned with ovulation and possibly causing a miscarriage; and that of men by causing erectile dysfunction, loss of libido and decreased sperm production. The advice is to find out about antidepressant drugs that will not affect fertility.

Antihistamine

These drugs are used for conditions such as hay fever and allergies. A common over-the-counter antihistamine is called Claritin. It may affect your fertility by drying cervical mucus, especially important if you monitor the changes to your cervical mucus to determine when ovulation occurs.

For men it may improve sperm quality. Always discuss medication with your healthcare professional as it is very important you don't self-medicate.

Anti-inflammatories

These are pain relief medication, also known as nonsteroidal anti-inflammatory drugs or NSAIDs, and are commonly prescribed for rheumatoid arthritis, back pain etc. They may affect fertility by preventing an egg being released from your ovary (ovulation) and by lowering progesterone hormone levels. Once you stop taking NSAIDs ovulation should return and your progesterone levels should return to normal.

Anti-Müllerian Hormone – AMH

This is a protein hormone produced by a type of cell within your ovaries and can be measured and tested at any time during your menstrual cycle. AMH is a blood test carried out to assess your supply of eggs, also known as your ovarian reserve. If you have this test you may be offered another test called an antral follicle count (AFC) scan. Some fertility professionals believe the AMH test is not as reliable as people think and the two tests together are better than the AMH on its own. The advice is that if you are told that you have low ovarian reserve and are trying to get pregnant, have regular sex. See 'Antral Follicle Count Scan' for more information.

If you have PCOS, your AMH levels are typically raised, so having this blood test is unlikely to be useful in predicating your egg reserve. Also, if you are doing IVF, it helps the doctor to decide on the dose of gonadotropin to give you and will help him/her to assess your risk of OHSS, see 'Ovarian/ovary Hyperstimulation Syndrome' for more information.

Anti-Nuclear Antibodies – ANA

Your body creates antibodies to help fight bacteria and germs that enter your body, and this is how you fight off infection, colds and other illnesses. In some people, their body mistakes normal cells for these invaders and anti-nuclear antibodies attack the nuclei (the centres) of these normal cells; as a result, inflammation and illness can occur. Small amounts of ANAs are normal and should not cause any complications. But, if you have large amounts of ANAs in your bloodstream, problems can occur because these antibodies destroy your healthy cells. Complications associated with ANAs include systemic lupus erythematosus (SLE), miscarriage and unexplained infertility.

Some fertility experts believe that if you have high levels of ANAs it causes inflammation in your uterus and placenta, contributing to miscarriage and implantation failure. Others believe there is no connection.

It should be noted that this is a very complicated area and everyone is different, so it is imperative that you seek the advice of a specialist rather than asking for advice on fertility forums.

Anti-Nuclear Antibody Test – ANA

This is a blood test that tests the levels of anti-nuclear antibodies or ANAs in your blood – see 'Anti-Nuclear Antibodies' (above) for more information. If you have high levels of ANAs in your blood further testing may be advised by your doctor. If the advice is to have treatment to help lower the levels, you may be prescribed a medication called prednisone/prednisolone, which is a steroid, and possibly aspirin. Your fertility doctor will discuss your results and any treatment with you.

Anti-ovarian Antibody – AOA, AVA

Antibodies are cells produced by your body to fight and destroy foreign bodies, such as those viruses and bacteria that cause colds and infection, and they help to make you better. Sometimes, your body gets confused and makes antibodies that fight against your own cells. Anti-ovarian antibodies are cells that damage your ovaries and eggs; as a consequence, they affect your ovulation and therefore your fertility.

AOAs are very often present in your bloodstream; small amounts are found in women who do not have fertility problems, but large amounts are usually in your blood if you have:

- premature ovarian failure (POF)
- unexplained infertility
- Addison's disease (disorder of your adrenal glands)
- thyroid problems
- endometriosis
- type 1 diabetes mellitus.

AOA are associated with:

- poor implantation
- poor hormone response
- IVF failure.

Your doctor may suggest you have a blood test to check the AOA levels in your blood if you are struggling to get pregnant. A sample of your blood will be sent to the lab and the results are either:

- negative – there are no antibodies in your blood
- positive – you have antibodies in your blood and this could be causing your fertility problems.

If you test positive, your doctor may prescribe medication that suppresses your immune system, with the aim of preventing your body from making AOAs.

Antioxidants

These protect the egg and sperm from free radical damage. Free radicals damage both cell health and the cell's DNA and could affect you from getting pregnant.

Anti-phospholipid Antibodies – APAs

These are proteins that are present in your bloodstream. They bind to cell membranes and make them sticky. This stops the blood from flowing properly and results in blood clots. There are twenty-one different types of APA and some experts believe high levels can cause the following:

- unexplained infertility
- miscarriage
- implantation failure
- IVF failure.

APAs are linked to recurrent miscarriage and if you have had three or more miscarriages before 12 weeks of pregnancy, or one or more miscarriages after 13 weeks but before 28 weeks of pregnancy, you should have one of the screening blood tests as it is one of the most treatable causes. With correct diagnosis and treatment, a majority of women have a successful pregnancy.

Anti-phospholipid Syndrome – APS

If you are tested and found to have anti-phospholipid antibodies (APAs) – see above, you will usually be diagnosed with anti-phospholipid syndrome, or APS, which is also known as Hughes syndrome or 'sticky blood'. If you have anti-phospholipid antibodies but do not have any symptoms or health problems, you would not be classed as having APS.

Anti-Sperm Antibodies

These occur in a condition that is sometimes called 'immunity to sperm' and is where the man's body attacks his sperm or your body attacks his sperm. Anti-sperm antibodies reduce fertility but do not prevent fertilisation. Antibodies are produced when sperm and blood come into contact (under normal conditions they don't), and occur following physical or chemical injury or infection, such as mumps. If high levels of antibodies are detected, the usual way forward to achieve a pregnancy is with ICSI.

The below is not to scale and is an artistic impression of a sperm.

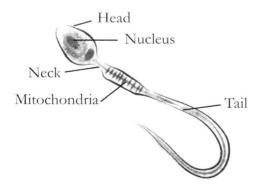

Anti-thyroid Antibodies

This is an autoimmune disorder where antibodies are directed against the thyroid gland and cause chronic inflammation. Over time, this results in the thyroid being unable to produce the correct levels of thyroid hormones which leads to a decline in functionality, and eventually an underactive thyroid (hypothyroidism). The presence of anti-thyroid antibodies is associated with an increased risk of unexplained infertility and miscarriage. See 'Hypothyroidism' for more information.

Antral Follicle Count scan – AFC

An antral follicle is a 'resting' follicle on your ovaries that contains an immature egg. A count of these follicles can be carried out by ultrasound, and together with an anti-Müllerian hormone (AMH) blood test, some fertility experts believe these tests can be highly effective in measuring your ovarian reserve, or how many immature eggs you have left in your ovaries. Others disagree.

You are born with your lifetime supply of eggs in your ovaries and as you age, fewer eggs remain and therefore there will be fewer antral follicles. See 'Anti-Müllerian Hormone' for more information.

Artificial Insemination – AI

This is more commonly known as intravaginal insemination; see this term for more information.

Asherman's Syndrome

This is a rare condition also known as intrauterine adhesions/ scarring or synechiae. It can occur if you have had several dilation and curettage (D&C) procedures causing adhesions or scar tissue to form inside your womb and/or cervix. In many cases the front and back walls of your womb stick to one another, or adhesions occur in a small area of your womb. The condition is classed as mild, moderate or severe depending on the extent of the adhesions.

Most women have scanty or no periods and it can affect your fertility by causing miscarriages or preventing an embryo from implanting in your endometrium or womb lining. The treatment is to have surgery to remove the adhesions – which unfortunately may cause more adhesions.

The below is not to scale and is an artistic impression of your reproductive system.

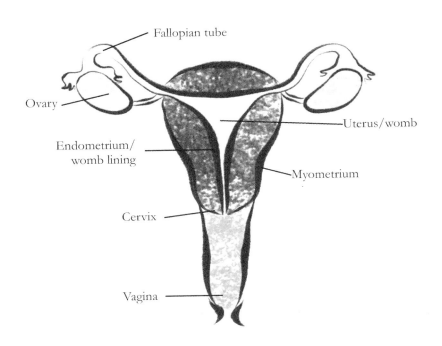

Assisted Hatching – AH

For an embryo to implant successfully into your womb lining it must first hatch out of its 'shell' (known as the zona pellucida or zona), so that the embryo cells come into direct contact with your womb lining cells. One reason for implantation failure during a natural conception or following IVF is that the embryo is unable to hatch because the shell surrounding the embryo is too hard or thick.

AH is a procedure that your clinic may offer, sometimes as an 'add-on' treatment during your IVF cycle, and it is carried out in the laboratory by an experienced embryologist who will make a hole in the shell using very small instruments or a laser. It is not thought that AH is necessary for everyone who is doing IVF but is thought to be of benefit:

• if you have poor quality embryos

• if you are older; more than 35, or in some countries 38

• if you have had two or more failed IVF cycles.

As with any treatment there are side effects, such as:

• damage to the embryo or cells resulting in an unsuccessful IVF cycle

• a higher risk of identical twins.

Assisted Reproductive Technology – ART

This is the technology used to achieve pregnancy in procedures such as fertility medication, artificial insemination, IVF and surrogacy. Also known as 'fertility treatments'.

Asthenospermia

Also called 'asthenozoospermia', this is the term for when a man has reduced sperm motility. 'Motility' is the sperm's ability to move forward, move quickly and in a straight line. If the motility of sperm is poor they're less likely to reach and fertilise an egg. This can be a cause of male factor infertility. Lifestyle changes could improve sperm abnormalities. See 'Sperm Motility' for more information.

Azoospermia – AZO/AZOO

This is when no sperm are found in a man's ejaculate. There are two types depending on what the cause is:

1. secretory azoospermia is when it is impossible for the testicles to produce sperm

2. obstructive azoospermia is when there is an obstruction between the testicles (where sperm are made) and the urethra, which releases sperm

The below is not to scale and is an artistic impression of the male reproductive system.

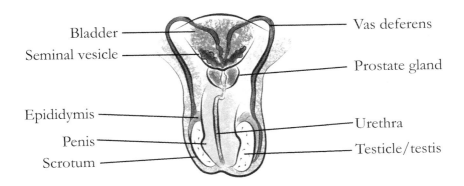

49

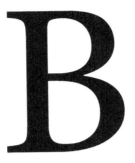

BABY DANCING

to

BREAKTHROUGH BLEEDING

A sperm cell measures about 0.05 mm from head to tail, whereas the egg cell measure 0.15-0.2 mm, i.e. about 30 times larger than the sperm and is just visible to the naked eye.

Baby Dancing – BD

A slang term for having unprotected sex with the intention of getting pregnant. Seen often on forums etc.

Bacterial Vaginosis – BV

This is when an abnormal level of bacteria is present in your vagina which changes the vaginal pH from acidic to alkaline. The cause is not known and the link between infertility and BV is not fully understood, but if you have BV you are more at risk of pelvic inflammatory disease (PID), which is a cause of infertility. You are more at risk of BV if you have multiple sexual partners, if you douche frequently and if you smoke, as these can upset the balance of bacteria.

You do not always experience symptoms, which is why it often goes untreated and leads to PID. If you do experience symptoms you may notice a watery discharge and a fishy odour from your vagina. Understandably if you have symptoms it can be quite distressing and embarrassing. It is not itchy so shouldn't be confused with thrush.

It is known that BV can be the cause of IVF being unsuccessful so it may be a good idea to be screened prior to starting any fertility treatment, even if it is just so you can tick it off the list.

Basal Body Temperature – BBT

This is your lowest body temperature when at rest, when you have been asleep for at least three hours. To get an accurate reading, it should be taken before any physical activity and before getting out of bed. When you ovulate your BBT increases by 0.5-1˚F, or 0.25-0.5˚C. See 'Basal Body Temperature Charting' (below) for more information on how your BBT can help you to get pregnant.

Basal Body Temperature Charting – BBTC

This is a useful and cheap way of finding out when/if you ovulate. You need to use a basal thermometer as this will accurately record the very small changes in temperature (read the reviews before you buy one as they do vary). You should take your temperature at the same time every morning and before you eat or drink. To work out when you ovulate you will need to record two or three menstrual cycles on a BBT chart – an example is over the page, and you can get one free from various fertility websites or use an app, of which there are many.

When you ovulate, hormonal changes cause your BBT to rise or 'spike' very slightly and to stay raised for the next three days. You are most fertile on the day of the temperature spike and on the few days before the spike, hence charting for at least two cycles, as you will then start to see a pattern and know which your best days are to have sex. BBT charting is most effective when you are also aware of the changes in your cervical mucus. See 'Cervical Mucus' for more information (With thanks to 'Your Fertility Self' for providing the following BBT chart).

Basal Body Temperature (BBT) and Cervical Mucus (CM) chart

Cycle Day	1	2	3	4	5	6	7	8	9	10	11	12	13	14	15	16	17	18	19	20	21	22	23	24	25	26	27	28	29	30	31
Date																															
Day of Week																															
Time Taken																															
Waking Temperature (°C)																															
36.9																															
36.8																															
36.7																															
36.6																															
36.5																															
36.4																															
36.3																															
36.2																															
36.1																															
36.0																															
35.9																															
Cycle Day	1	2	3	4	5	6	7	8	9	10	11	12	13	14	15	16	17	18	19	20	21	22	23	24	25	26	27	28	29	30	31
Bleeding																															
CM																															
Cervix (hard/soft)																															
Cervix Position (high/low)																															
OPK Result (+/-)																															
Intercourse?																															
Comments (e.g., poor sleep, ill, alcohol)																															

Key: Bleeding: S=Slight, M=Moderate, H=Heavy, C=Clots   CM: D=Dry, W=Wet, S=Sticky, EWCM=Egg White

Beta hCG Pregnancy Test – Beta

This is a blood test to detect the presence of the pregnancy hormone hCG (human chorionic gonadotropin). There are two tests – a qualitative test and a quantitative test/ beta hCG:

1. The qualitative test will give you a 'yes' or 'no' answer similar to what you get with a home pregnancy test (HPT) when you pee on a stick.

2. A quantitative test/beta provides the amount of hCG in your blood and is useful if you have had fertility treatment or have a history of miscarriages. Knowing the level of hCG means you will know if the level is increasing with further blood tests. Typically, hCG levels double every 48 to 72 hours in an early healthy pregnancy. Clinics generally ask you to have this test done after fertility treatment so they know the level of hCG.

If you have had IVF, ICSI or any variation of these, your clinic will ask you to have a blood test 9-12 days after your embryo transfer; nine days if you had a five-day blastocyst transfer, 11 days if you had a three-day embryo transfer and 12 days if you had a two-day embryo transfer. This is to hopefully ensure that all the hCG from the trigger shot is out of your bloodstream. The general guideline is that it takes one day per 1,000 units of hCG trigger shot to leave your blood, so if you had 10,000 units of hCG, it should all be out of your bloodstream by Day 10. But we are all different so it's best to be cautious and test when your clinic tells you to – if you have the test too early you may get an incorrect result, which you really don't want.

If your hCG level is less than 5 mIU/mL (milli-interational units/ millilitre) unfortunately this means you are not pregnant. If the level is between 6-24 mIU/mL it means you might be pregnant so you will be asked to have the test done again in 48 hours to check that the level has increased. If your hCG level is 25 mIU/mL, this indicates a positive pregnancy test.

Big Fat Negative – BFN

The abbreviation for when you get a dreaded negative pregnancy result, either from a home pregnancy test (HPT) or a blood test.

Big Fat Positive – BFP

The abbreviation for when you get a much-wanted positive pregnancy result, either from a home pregnancy test (HPT) or a blood test.

Birth Control Pills – BCP

Also called oral contraceptive pills or simply 'The Pill'. They are medications that prevent pregnancy. They are either combinations of the hormones oestrogen and progestin known as the combined oral contraceptive pill, or they are progestin only (synthethic form of progesterone). The combined pill works by preventing the release of two hormones, luteinising hormone (LH) and follicle-stimulating hormone (FSH) from the pituitary gland in the brain. These two hormones are necessary for the development of the egg and the preparation on your womb lining for implantation of an embryo. Progestin also acts on the mucus that surrounds the egg making it more difficult for a sperm to penetrate it.

Bisphenol A – BPA

This is a chemical that is often used to manufacture hard plastic products, such as water bottles, microwave-safe food containers and the lining of aluminium cans. Studies have suggested that its presence in water and foods can affect sperm count, egg quality and quantity and may be linked to polycystic ovary/ovarian syndrome, or PCOS. When buying food/drink storage products, look for those that are 'BPA free' or use glass or china to store or reheat food.

Blighted Ovum – BO

This is when a fertilised egg attaches to the wall of your womb but an embryo doesn't develop. Cells develop forming the pregnancy sac but not an embryo. It occurs within the first 12 weeks of pregnancy and often it's so early, at five to six weeks, that you don't even know you're pregnant. A blighted ovum often occurs due to chromosomal problems or abnormal cell division. There is nothing you could have done to prevent it and it's important to know that it is not your fault.

Blocked Fallopian Tubes

A Fallopian tube is a very narrow tube that links your ovary to your womb and carries a mature egg to your womb during your menstrual cycle. Normally you have two ovaries and hence two tubes lying either side of your womb. One or both tubes may become blocked which may make it difficult for the sperm to reach your egg and for the fertilised egg to reach your womb. The tubes can be blocked totally or partially and if partially blocked, this can cause an ectopic or 'tubal' pregnancy.

Often you don't experience any symptoms, though sometimes blocked tubes can lead to other medical conditions such as endometriosis and pelvic inflammatory disease (PID). Hydrosalpinx is when you do get symptoms – for example, lower abdominal pain and vaginal discharge. Other causes of blocked tubes are:

- pelvic inflammatory disease or PID
- chlamydia in the past or currently
- uterine infection
- previous ectopic pregnancy
- abdominal surgery
- endometriosis.

57

You may find out you have a blocked tube or tubes during a hysterosalpingogram (HSG), an investigation carried out because you can't get pregnant. Other tests may include an ultrasound, exploratory laparoscopic surgery or blood tests for chlamydia. If you have one blocked tube there is a good chance that you can get pregnant (if there are no other causes to you not getting pregnant), and you may be given fertility drugs to increase ovulation on the side of the open tube. If both tubes are blocked, a laparoscopy will be carried out to try and remove adhesions and scar tissue, but there is no guarantee that this will be successful. If this is the case then you would need to discuss treatments such as IVF with your doctor. The below is not to scale and is an artistic impression of a blocked Fallopian tube.

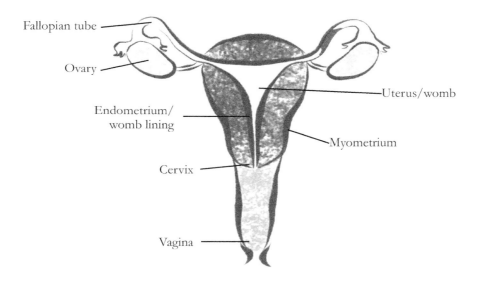

Blood Test/Work – BW, b/w

There are many blood tests that you may have to have done in order to find out why you are struggling to get pregnant. They are more often than not checking the level of certain hormones on certain days of your menstrual cycle. I have listed them below but each one can be found in this book if you want to find out more information.

They are:

- cortisol
- follicle-stimulating hormone (FSH)
- luteinising hormone (LH)
- oestrogen/estrogen
- progesterone
- prolactin
- rubella
- sex hormone binding globulin (SHBG)
- testosterone
- thyroid
- thyroid stimulating hormone (TSH)
- T3 and T4 levels
- vitamins B12, B6 and D
- zinc.

There are also some blood tests that the man should have done, namely:

- Male hormone profile which includes LH, FSH, TSH, T3 and T4 levels, testosterone, SHBG and prolactin
- It may also be a good idea that he has his levels of folate, vitamins B12, B6 and D and zinc checked.

There are a couple of blood tests that your doctor may also carry out that are not to do with finding out the cause of your struggle to get pregnant, but are done to protect your baby should you get pregnant, and they are:

- folate

- rubella

- cytomegalovirus (CMV)

All these are explained in further detail in this book.

Body Mass Index – BMI

This is an index of your skinniness or heaviness and it factors in your weight and height to give an overall index. Your weight, whether extremely thin or obese, can affect your fertility because the normal process of regular, consistent ovulation may be disrupted. It isn't perfect because there are other things that should be considered when it comes to your weight, but it is used as a guide by fertility specialists.

You work out your BMI by dividing your weight by your height then divide your answer by your height again. For example, if you weigh 60 kgs (9 st 6 lbs) and you are 1.7 m (5 ft 5 in) tall, your BMI is worked out like this: 60 divided by 1.7 (= 35.29) and divide by 1.7 again = a BMI of 20.75 kg/m2.

As with practically everything to do with fertility, you will get varying answers from doctors, lay people and websites as to what range is 'normal'. As a rough guide, a healthy BMI score is between 18.5 and 25. If your score is under 18.5 this indicates that you are underweight. If your score is 25.1-29.9 this indicates that you are 'overweight', but not obese. If your score is over 30 this indicates you are 'obese' and a score of over 40 indicates you are 'extremely obese'.

In the UK, the clinical commissioning groups or CCGs consider your weight and BMI if you are applying for funding for fertility treatment.

Breakthrough Bleeding – BTB

Sometimes called 'spotting', this is bleeding during your menstrual cycle (not to be confused with your period). It can be caused by there not being enough of the hormone oestrogen/estrogen.

British Fertility Society

This was founded in 1972 by a small group with a common interest in infertility. Today, the society recognises the multidisciplinary nature of reproductive medicine and welcomes doctors, andrologists, counsellors, embryologists, endocrinologists, nurses and other professional groups working in this field into its membership.

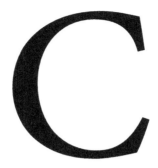

CANCELLED CYCLE

to

CYTOMEGALOVIRUS – CMV

On average, IVF fails 70% of the time. (HFEA)

Cancelled Cycle

This is when an ART cycle such as IVF is stopped before egg collection or, in the case of a frozen embryo cycle, before the embryo(s) is transferred. The reasons a cycle may be cancelled are numerous but include:

- undeveloped eggs
- an endometrial lining that is too thin
- you become ill
- frozen embryo hasn't thawed properly.

It is extremely upsetting if your cycle has to be cancelled due to events that are out of your control. Your clinic will only cancel a cycle if it is unavoidable. It is very important that you talk about why it is cancelled with your doctor or nurse and understand that it is not your fault. If you struggle to accept that your cycle has been cancelled (and this is not uncommon), you may find it helps to speak to a counsellor or a fertility coach.

Cervical Mucus – CM

This is a vaginal discharge that changes in amount, texture and colour during your menstrual cycle, due to an increase in your oestrogen levels. You can monitor and record these changes to help you know when you are ovulating. It may also help if you record your basal body temperature (BBT) at the same time – see 'Basal Body Temperature Charting' for more information.

This is how your CM changes during your menstrual cycle:

- during your period you lose menstrual blood
- after the bleeding has finished your CM may be dry for several days, or it may be cloudy coloured, similar to the consistency of sticky rice; it's very unlikely that you would

conceive whilst your CM is like this

- then your CM becomes clear and slippery and it increases in volume, becoming more like raw egg white in colour and consistency (often referred to as 'egg white cervical mucus' or EWCM) as you enter your fertile window – the time you will most likely conceive if you have unprotected sex. This slippery mucus will make it easier for sperm to reach your egg. If you are doing fertility treatment such as IVF, it's not uncommon to produce more EWCM than usual. Don't panic (like I did when we did our first IVF round) that you are about to ovulate before your egg collection/retrieval – you won't because of the medication you are taking.

- roughly three days after this fertile mucus starts, clear mucus strings may appear. In the next day or two, your CM becomes even wetter and more slippery – you are at your most fertile when it reaches a peak of wetness and slipperiness

- once you have reached your peak day, your CM becomes dry or cloudy and sticky once more. This change for two or more consecutive days means that your fertile window has now passed.

Charting your CM is very quick and easy and consists of you checking daily to see if your mucus is fertile or not. You can choose to record your findings on a chart you have downloaded from a website or use a mobile phone app. Do some research on apps to find the right one for yourself as they do vary.

Cervical Position – CP

The position (and texture) of the cervix changes during your menstrual cycle and you can monitor the changes, together with the changes in your cervical mucus and basal body temperature (BBT), to find out when your fertile window is. When your period has finished, the cervix is low and hard but as you approach ovulation, it moves to the top of the vagina and is softer and moister.

Cervical Stenosis

This is when the opening to the cervix is narrower than it should be or it is completely closed. This may cause infertility in the following ways:

- if completely closed, sperm cannot swim through to reach an egg to fertilise it

- if your menstrual blood cannot flow out it may cause your womb to become inflamed and infected and it could cause endometriosis

- the production of your cervical mucus may be less if the stenosis is due to scar tissue, which would result in the sperm having trouble moving and surviving.

During fertility treatment such as IVF or IUI, a thin, plastic tube or catheter is used to transfer the embryo or sperm into your womb. The catheter has to be passed through your cervix and if your cervix is narrow or closed, this makes it difficult. This is why your clinic may carry out a 'mock transfer' or 'trial of transfer' when you are doing fertility treatment, just to check there won't be any problems with your embryo transfer.

Cervix

Also called the neck of the uterus, this is the lower, narrow part that joins to the top of the vagina. The opening of the cervix is called the 'os' and it is through the os that your menstrual blood flows out of and into the vagina during menstruation, and sperm swim through during sex to reach an egg in order to fertilise it. The below is not to scale and is an artistic impression of your reproductive system.

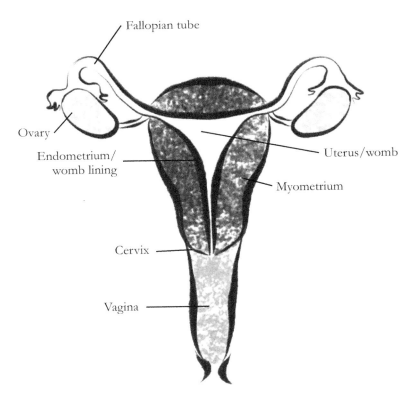

Chemical Pregnancy – CP

This is described as a very early miscarriage occurring before the fifth week of pregnancy and well before the baby would be detected by ultrasound. You may only know you've had a chemical pregnancy because you had a positive early pregnancy test but then tested again and it was negative, or your period was a week late.

It is believed they occur because the fertilised egg had chromosomal abnormalities. The reason for a positive pregnancy test is because, although the embryo didn't actually implant, the cells of the fertilised egg still produced enough of the pregnancy hormone hCG (human chorionic gonadotropin) to be detected by a pregnancy test.

Sheila says: Please be reassured that we all react differently and there is no right or wrong way as to how you should feel if you have a chemical pregnancy. If you are really devastated and feel you have lost your baby don't let anyone tell you otherwise. Grieve as you would for any loss and seek support from a miscarriage charity, or from someone you know who has also suffered a miscarriage and who is OK to support and talk to you. Do not bottle it up as it could affect you in so many ways in the future – post-traumatic stress disorder (PTSD) has been associated with women who have had a miscarriage. Other people you are close to, like your partner or family, may also be grieving.

Even after we were successful following our third ICSI cycle and our daughter was a toddler, I still cried when I thought about our baby we had lost at five to six weeks after our second ICSI cycle, and I couldn't understand why, until I was diagnosed years later with PTSD.

Chemotherapy

If you are having or will need to have chemotherapy because of cancer, it can affect your fertility. If you want to consider preserving your fertility so that you can have a family in the future, it is possible. You will need to speak to your doctor or cancer team about your options. The UK charity Cancer.org states: 'Studies have suggested that women with cancer are less likely to be given information about preserving their fertility than men.' This means you may need to bring up the subject with your doctor.

Currently your options are: freezing embryos, freezing eggs and freezing ovarian tissue.

Most chemotherapy drugs can damage your eggs but some drugs have a lower risk than others – again, seek the advice from the team who are caring for you.

Chicago Blood Tests

These are several blood tests that you might choose to have done following unsuccessful ART when the cause for your infertility is not known. The name comes from a doctor called Alan Beer from the US, who studied over many years the relationship between fertility, autoimmune and blood clotting issues. This area is very controversial and there are fertility clinics who do not offer the tests as they don't believe they help you to get pregnant, and there are other clinics who can organise the tests and give the treatment.

Chinese Herbs

They have been used to treat many health conditions, including fertility issues, for over 2,000 years. They are often used in conjunction with other Chinese medicine, especially acupuncture. Why Chinese herbs are believed to help with fertility issues is because they provide your body with nutrients and help to restore and rebalance it. Once balance is achieved, your chances of getting pregnant could improve.

Any type of fertility issue can be treated with Chinese herbs, including:

- luteal-phase deficit (LPD)
- premature ovarian failure (POF)
- advanced maternal age (AMA)
- unexplained infertility
- sperm issues, such as low sperm count.

If you decide to take herbs you will likely have to take them for several months, although if they are being taken to improve sperm, it is likely to be three months of treatment. It is so important that you do not self-prescribe and take herbs that you have bought off the internet. You must do your research and work with a practitioner who is certified (each country where Chinese medicine is practised will have their own certification). If you are wanting to use herbs in conjunction with fertility treatment such as IVF, you must tell your fertility clinic. Some may be more open to the idea than others but if you don't ask, you won't know.

Chlamydia

This bacterial infection can affect women and men and cause infertility in both sexes. If you have had chlamydia and it is not treated with antibiotics, it can spread to your womb, ovaries and/or Fallopian tubes and cause pelvic inflammatory disease or PID.

If a man isn't treated for chlamydia, it can spread to the testicles and epididymis (the tubes that carry sperm from the testicles), and it may cause infertility.

Chromosomes

These are found inside each cell of animals and plants and contain our DNA. Chromosomes occur in pairs and we have 23 pairs; other animals and plants have different numbers of pairs. They are in pairs because one set comes from the egg and the other set from the sperm.

Cleaved Embryo

This is an embryo at Day 2 or 3 after egg collection. Its cells are dividing (or 'cleaving') but the embryo doesn't grow in size yet. It is common for the embryologist to note that the embryo has three, five or six cells and this indicates the embryo is growing normally.

Please note: the illustration below is not to scale nor accurate with regard to embryo grading; it is more to give you a bit of an idea of what a developing embryo from Day 2 to Day 5 looks like.

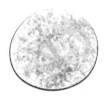
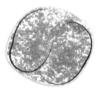
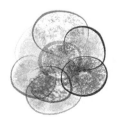
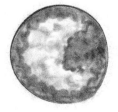

Clinical Pregnancy

This is when your pregnancy is confirmed by hCG (human chorionic gonadotropin), commonly called the 'pregnancy hormone', being detected in a pregnancy test and the gestational sac being visible on an ultrasound scan. The embryo itself may not actually be seen if the ultrasound is performed very early on because it is so small.

Sheila says: An early scan is one of the most wonderful things you will ever see in your pregnancy. Nothing beats seeing your tiny baby or babies so early on in his/her/their development. It's especially precious if you have struggled to get to this stage.

Clomid/Clomiphene

Clomid is the brand name of a drug given as fertility treatment to help you ovulate if you do not develop and release an egg naturally. It is taken as a tablet and usually you start taking it on Day 3 or Day 5 of your menstrual cycle – which exact day depends on your fertility doctor. You then take it for five days, and during this period you will be monitored by ultrasound and blood tests to check how many follicles are growing and when you ovulate. You will then be advised when is the best time to have sex. If too many follicles grow you will be advised to not have sex as this could result in a multiple pregnancy.

Clomid is often prescribed if you have polycystic ovarian/ovary syndrome (PCOS). See 'Polycystic Ovarian/Ovary Syndrome' for more information.

Clomiphene citrate may be given to men who have a low sperm count as taking the drug every day for a period of time can increase the production of sperm. A few weeks after he starts to take the drug, his testosterone hormone level will be checked to ensure he is not over-responding.

Compassionate Transfer

Following successful ART, years later when you have completed your family you may need to decide as to what happens to any remaining frozen embryos you have. There are a number of options and this is one of them, and it is when the remaining embryos are transferred back into your womb when it is unlikely to result in a pregnancy. This feels more natural to some people than any of the other options, which are donating to research, donating to another woman/couple or being destroyed.

Comprehensive Chromosome Screening

This screening may be carried out during IVF or similar fertility treatments, especially if you are:

- 35 years old or older

- have had previous failed IVF cycles

- have had recurrent miscarriages

- have had a previous pregnancy with a chromosomal abnormality.

The screening procedure is carried out by removing cells from the embryo whilst it is developing in the laboratory, and the number of chromosomes is measured. If the embryo has too many or too few chromosomes this can cause implantation failure or a miscarriage, and that embryo would not be selected for transfer. Babies conceived naturally with the incorrect number of chromosomes can have genetic conditions that are often life threatening.

Cortisol

This is a hormone, along with the hormone adrenaline, that is released from your adrenal glands in response to stress. Your adrenal glands sit on top of your kidneys. Stress is one of nature's contraceptives and can have a dramatic effect on healthy reproduction. Cortisol is derived from progesterone, which is essential for fertility, mainly through implantation of a fertilised egg and thickening of the lining of your womb each month. High levels of cortisol also prevent production of the main sex hormone GnRH (gonadotropin-releasing hormone), which in turn suppresses ovulation and sperm count. Diets that are high in stimulants and sugar drive cortisol levels up and therefore disrupt levels of your reproductive hormones. Most of us do not get enough sleep, so to wake ourselves up we need stimulants like sugar and coffee – this helps with your energy levels but is not helpful to your fertility. See 'Stress' for more information.

You can have your cortisol level checked by having a blood test and this is advisable if you are struggling to get pregnant.

Crosshairs – CH

The lines drawn on your basal body temperature chart to indicate ovulation. See 'Basal Body Temperature Charting' for more information.

Cryopreservation

This is the freezing of cells, such as eggs/oocytes, in liquid nitrogen at -196 °C, to preserve them for future use. See 'Egg Freezing' and 'Embryo Freezing' for more information.

Culture Medium

Once eggs are collected during ART, they are hopefully fertilised by a sperm and they begin to develop and grow. As they are not in your womb, the fertilised eggs are placed in a plastic dish that has a substance in it called 'culture medium'. This culture is made up of proteins, salts, sugars, water and nutrients, and it is this that supports and feeds the embryo until it is transferred back into your womb.

Cycle day – CD

A day in your menstrual cycle. Certain events happen on particular days during your cycle and if these are out of synch you may have issues with getting pregnant.

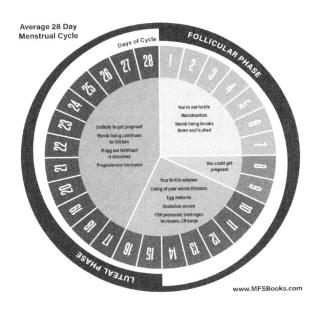

Cycle Day 1 – CD1

Either referring to the first day of your menstrual cycle or the first day of your IVF or fertility treatment cycle.

Cycle Number – CY#

This refers to the number of ART cycles you have done, so 'CY#3' means you have done three cycles or rounds of, for example, IVF.

Cytomegalovirus – CMV

This is a type of herpes virus transmitted from person to person via bodily fluids, typically in saliva but also urine, blood, vaginal secretions and semen. The only symptoms that you have it are similar to a common cold:

- fever
- achy muscles and joints
- sore throat
- swollen glands, etc.

Once you've had CMV, the virus remains in your body but you have no symptoms unless your immune system is compromised by stress or another infection so isn't working as efficiently as it should.

CMV can also be spread from a pregnant mother to her unborn baby if it is contracted for the first time while the baby is in your womb. It is the most commonly transmitted virus to developing babies and can cause:

- deafness
- blindness
- microcephaly (smaller than normal head)
- organ failure
- cognitive developmental delays (the process of acquiring and understanding knowledge through thoughts, experiences and the senses).

Your baby is not at risk if you caught the CMV virus before you got pregnant. You can have a blood test to check for antibodies prior to trying to get pregnant.

If you are considering using a sperm donor, from somewhere other than a sperm bank, it would be wise to check that the donor didn't have CMV when he donated the sperm.

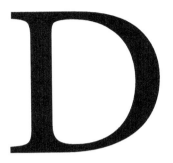

DEHYDROEPIANDROSTERONE to DOWN REGULATION

The follicle-stimulating hormone (FSH) and luteinsing hormone (LH) that is in medication used for fertility treatment traditionally came from the urine of nuns in Italy and was known as 'human menopausal gonadotropins' or hMG.

Dehydroepiandrosterone – DHEA

This is a natural steroid hormone produced in your adrenal glands (located on top of your kidneys). DHEA levels peak when you reach the age of 25 and then steadily decline as you get older. DHEA is made into supplements made from soy or wild yam roots.

Regarding fertility, some health practitioners believe it helps improve egg health in women over 40 and helps if you have low ovarian reserve (LOR) or premature ovarian failure (POF), whilst others believe there is little evidence to support this. Because our bodies are not supposed to have high levels of DHEA as we age, in the long run it may cause hormonal imbalances.

It is very important that DHEA supplements are only taken on the advice of your health practitioner; never self-prescribe. Side effects can include oily skin, headache, nausea and mood changes.

Diagnosis – Dx

This is when a judgement about what a particular illness is, is made after examining your symptoms. You need a diagnosis in order for your doctor to treat you accordingly.

Dilation & Curettage – D&C

This is a short surgical procedure, so called because during it your cervix is dilated or expanded in order to scrape your womb lining, or endometrium, with a curette (a spoon-shaped surgical instrument). You will probably feel some pain and cramping afterwards but it doesn't usually last longer than 24 hours. Bleeding lasts from a few days up to a couple of weeks. It is carried out to diagnose and treat certain uterine conditions, such as heavy bleeding.

Dilation & Evacuation – D&E

If, unfortunately you have a miscarriage called a 'missed miscarriage', it means that some of the baby remains inside your womb. This can cause you to continue to have pregnancy symptoms and to also continue to bleed for longer than is usual. This is dangerous to you as you could get an infection, so you may have a procedure called a D&E (also called an ERPC – evacuation of retained products of conception – a horrible word I know). It is carried out in the same way as a D&C, explained above.

Diminished Ovarian Reserve – DOR

The current belief is that as you age, so do your eggs. DOR is when there is a decrease in the number of eggs, which are insufficient to ensure a reasonable chance of pregnancy. The first sign is long menstrual cycles and infrequent periods. It usually occurs around menopause and the age we reach the menopause varies for each of us. See 'Low Ovarian Reserve' for more information.

Donor Egg – DE

This is an egg used during fertility treatment, such as IVF or ICSI, that is from another woman, who may or may not be related to you. You may decide to use a donor egg in order to have a baby for the following reasons:

- your ovaries are not producing any eggs
- you have done a number of IVF/ICSI cycles etc that have not resulted in you having a baby
- your own eggs are considered 'old'
- you have unexplained infertility
- you are a carrier of a life-threatening illness.

For many this is a very difficult decision to make, for others it isn't difficult; everyone is different and no one decision is right or wrong. You may be afraid that you won't bond with your baby or that the baby won't look like you. For some couples, the man may not want to use donor eggs because he feels the baby won't be part of you and he is worried he won't be able to love it because of this. All these are perfectly normal fears and feelings.

Any baby born to you, or both of you, from a donated egg will absolutely, totally be your baby; you will have carried him or her for nine months, you will have fed and protected your baby, you will have felt them move and seen them grow, they have heard your voice(s). Do not let anyone tell you that the baby is not yours.

How much information you know about your donor varies from country to country as does the cost; in some countries donors only receive a payment for their expenses whereas in other countries donors are paid thousands. You also need to consider whether you prefer the donor to be anonymous or not; if the donor is anonymous, any children born to you from the donation will not be able to contact the donor in the future; or, when they reach 18 years old, they can find out the donor's name and last known address.

By law in the UK you must be offered implications counselling to ensure you have considered fully what it means to have a donor-conceived child. See 'Egg Donor' for more information.

Donor Egg In Vitro Fertilisation – DE IVF

A donor egg is fertilised with your partner's sperm or sperm from a donor during an IVF cycle. As with a standard IVF cycle, the embryos are allowed to develop and usually one is transferred into your womb where it will hopefully implant successfully, and you will carry your baby until s/he is born. See 'Egg Donor' for more information.

Donor Insemination – DI

Also known as 'artificial insemination', this is when a man (the donor) provides sperm in a sperm sample and the sperm is used to fertilise your egg. The fertilisation may occur by you inseminating yourself or doing IUI at a fertility clinic.

DI is carried out when there is:

- the absence of a male partner
- poor quality sperm
- no sperm
- genetic disorders that could be passed onto any children.

The below is not to scale and is purely an artistic impression of the DI procedure.

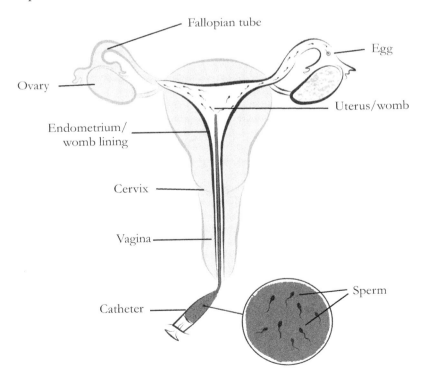

Fallopian tube

Egg

Ovary

Uterus/womb

Endometrium/ womb lining

Cervix

Vagina

Sperm

Catheter

Double Embryo Transfer – DET

This is where two embryos are transferred back into your womb following IVF, ICSI or intracytoplasmic morphologically selected sperm injection (IMSI) and can therefore lead to twins or triplets. Transferring two embryos is usually at the discretion of the fertility clinic. Some countries do not carry out a DET; they will only transfer one embryo. See 'Elective Single Embryo Transfer' for more information.

Down Regulation

This is part of the procedure when you are doing IVF or similar fertility treatment, and it is the first step you will go through as it shuts down the pituitary-ovarian hormones, which has the effect of preventing premature ovulation. This is also known as 'suppression'.

In your natural menstrual cycle, when the dominant follicle has reached a certain size, your oestrogen is at a specific level that tells the pituitary gland to release a surge of luteinising hormone (LH) which brings about ovulation. However, in IVF for example, as you have a number of follicles growing, your oestrogen levels will reach the specific level for your pituitary gland to release the surge of LH too soon; therefore, premature ovulation would occur before your egg collection/retrieval, which you definitely don't want.

The medication that you will be prescribed to prevent premature ovulation is known as a gonadotropin-releasing hormone or GnRH. You will take the medication either as a nasal spray, or as a once-a-day injection. Try not to worry about having to do injections, you will be shown at the clinic and if you really can't, ask your partner or a good friend to help you.

You start taking the medication on Day 2 or Day 21 depending on whether you are following a short or long protocol. For your ovaries to be completely suppressed takes approximately two weeks. You will have an ultrasound scan to confirm all is going as it should and the ultrasound will show a thin uterine lining and 'sleeping' ovaries. A blood test to check the hormone level of oestradiol is also carried out to confirm suppression.

Some side effects you may experience are:

- hot flushes/flashes
- headache
- nausea
- weight gain
- bruising/rash at injection sites.

The next stage after down regulation is your ovaries are stimulated to produce more follicles and therefore more mature eggs. See 'Stimulation' for more information.

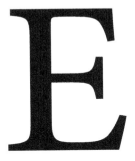

EARLY PREGNANCY SYMPTOMS

to

EUROPEAN SOCIETY OF
HUMAN REPRODUCTION AND
EMBRYOLOGY

Infertility is caused by the female in one-third of cases and
the male in one-third of cases. The remainder are caused
by a mixture of male and female issues or the cause is not
known. (From RESOLVE in the US)

Early Morning Urine – EMU

See 'First Morning Urine' for more information.

Early Pregnancy Symptoms

The most important thing to remember when your period is about due or during your two-week wait (TWW) is that every woman is different, and if you don't think you have any symptoms associated with pregnancy, then this does not mean you are not pregnant. If you search online for this term you will read all sorts of symptoms from the weird to the wonderful; which is another reason not to search on a certain famous website (but I know you'll want to). Even your friends who have got pregnant naturally will either experience none, some or all of the early symptoms.

It is very important to remember that you have taken loads of hormonal drugs in the last weeks or months, your womb and ovaries have been prodded and poked, and you have been so focused on eggs and womb lining that it's hardly surprising that you are now analysing every single twinge and emotion and feeling.

Here are some symptoms that you may experience or you may not:

- spotting or light bleeding isn't an indication necessarily that your period is about to start – it could be your embryo implanting; however, if you don't have any spotting it may be that you didn't notice any rather than you haven't had any

- mild cramping in your tummy area is normal and is due to the prodding and poking that has been going on in that area; if it is severe contact your clinic

- sore and bigger boobs are caused by the hormone progesterone which you will be taking during your TWW

- feeling sick or being sick
- tiredness, caused by a huge surge of progesterone
- backache.

Remember, that the only way to confirm whether you are pregnant or not is to do a home pregnancy test (HPT) or a blood test.

Ectopic Pregnancy – EP

This is when the fertilised egg implants outside of your womb, usually in the Fallopian tube, and in rare cases the cervix or an ovary. It is also known as 'tubal pregnancy'. It is only very slightly more likely to happen after fertility treatment, such as IVF, than in a natural pregnancy.

Common symptoms of an ectopic pregnancy are:

- bleeding
- nausea and vomiting with pain
- sharp cramps in your abdomen
- dizziness
- pain in your shoulder, neck or back passage.

If untreated it can rupture your Fallopian tube and this is an emergency, so if you get any of the above symptoms, you must seek medical help. It may result in surgery and in some cases, your Fallopian tube may have to be removed.

Egg/Oocyte/Ovum

The medical term for 'egg' is oocyte or ovum (the plural is ova), but egg is what we tend to say mostly. It is the largest cell in your body and is about the size of a grain of sand, about 0.12mm in diameter, so you can actually see it with your naked eye. Amazing.

You start making your eggs (or egg cells) nine weeks after you are conceived, and you'll have made around seven million by the time you are 20 weeks old – that's while you're still inside your mum's womb. By the time you are born, you'll only have around two million eggs as a massive number will have died. Approximately 1,000 die every month, that's 30-35 every day, and you ovulate around 400-500 eggs in your lifetime. It has always been believed that you won't make any more eggs; however, scientists recently discovered a new type of stem cell in a woman's ovary that suggest the possibility of new eggs continually being produced throughout our reproductive years.

There are four parts to an egg cell: nucleus, cytoplasm, zona pellucinda and corona radiata.

1. The nucleus is the heart of the egg and contains the 23 chromosomes. The genes are also found here.

2. The cytoplasm is a gel-like substance and it is here that all the cell's activities take place to keep it alive and functioning properly. This is where the mitochondria are – these supply most of the energy for the egg.

3. The zona pellucida is the egg wall (a little like an eggshell), and it helps the sperm to enter the egg for fertilisation to happen. The egg wall hardens with age.

4. The corona radiata consists of two or three layers of cells from the follicle and surrounds the egg. They are attached to the zona pellucida and their main function is to supply vital proteins to the egg.

When you are 21 years old, about 90% of your eggs are viable, meaning they would be fertilised if they met with a sperm. At 41 years old, only about 10% of your eggs might be viable. At age 37 years, you have about 25,000 eggs and after 37/38 years of age the number of eggs that die every month rapidly increases.

During your menstrual cycle you usually only ovulate one egg, though sometimes each ovary releases an egg during ovulation and this is called 'hyper-ovulation', which could result in non-identical twins if both eggs are fertilised. The reasons for this happening naturally are when there is a family history on the mother's side or if you have PCOS.

Once an egg has matured and is released from the ovary during ovulation, the egg is wafted by hair-like projections called 'cilia' into the Fallopian tube where it waits for a sperm. But it's quite impatient and only lives for between 12 and 24 hours. If sperm is already in your Fallopian tube when ovulation occurs or very soon after, the egg is more likely to be fertilised. When an egg is fertilised by a sperm, it releases special proteins and enzymes to ensure another sperm doesn't get in. The fertilised egg is then moved down your Fallopian tube by the cilia until it reaches your womb some six-plus days later, when it will hopefully implant in the lining of your womb. Also see 'Egg Quality' for more information.

The below is not to scale and is an artistic impression of your egg.

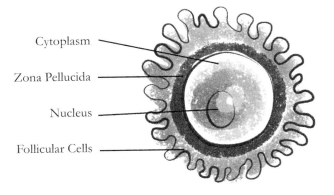

Cytoplasm

Zona Pellucida

Nucleus

Follicular Cells

Egg Bank

This is a storage facility for eggs donated by women in order to help another woman, or a couple or a surrogate, to get pregnant. If you are doing donor egg in vitro fertilisation (DE IVF) then your clinic may go to an egg bank to find you a donor if they do not get the donor themselves. See 'Egg Donor' for more information.

Egg Collection/Retrieval – EC/ER

This is one of the most dreaded but also most exciting days when you are doing fertility treatment such as IVF, because now you find out how many eggs your ovaries have produced whilst you've been doing ghastly injections and having moods swings a teenager would be proud of.

You usually go into the clinic in the morning after a phone call the day before. This day is classed as Day 0. You may have a general anaesthetic or sedation where you remain conscious. The usual collection method is done vaginally under sedation using an ultrasound. However, if one or both ovaries are difficult to get to this way, it will be done via your tummy using a procedure called a laparoscopy.

The procedure for vaginal collection is as follows (though how they actually collect the eggs is similar whichever procedure you have). It's similar to a smear/pap smear in that a vaginal probe is inserted into your vagina with a needle attached to the end that will collect the egg and fluid from the follicles in the ovaries. The ultrasound guides the doctor. Fluid is collected from each follicle and then passed to the embryologist who identifies, using a microscope, if there is an egg in the fluid. If there is no egg, the follicle is flushed with a solution and sucked out. If an egg is identified, the doctor repeats the procedure in the next follicle in the same ovary until all follicles are empty. The doctor then moves the needle to the other ovary and repeats the collection from each follicle.

You can go home after your EC/ER and you'll probably feel sore and in some pain from all the prodding and poking for a couple of days, so it's a good idea to have a couple of days chilling and relaxing if at all possible.

At the same time as you are having your EC/ER, your partner, if you are using his sperm, will be providing the sperm. The clinic prepares his sperm, or the donated sperm if you are using sperm donation.

After the egg collection a member of staff will confirm with you the number of eggs that were collected, the quality of the sperm sample and how the eggs will be fertilised, by IVF, ICSI or intracytoplasmic morphologically selected sperm injection (IMSI). You will also be told when a member of staff will contact you to let you know how many eggs have fertilised and other important information about contact from the clinic and any medication you still need to take.

Sheila says: Very exciting but very nerve wracking and everyone feels different around this time of their cycle. When we did our first IVF cycle, after EC until the embryo was transferred, it felt like I had lost something so precious and I was constantly deeply anxious and upset. I wanted to sit by the incubator my eggs were in and not take my eyes off them and metaphorically hold their hands, willing them to develop into our babies. It was a very strange feeling, nothing like I had experienced before.

The below is not to scale and is purely an artistic impression of the egg collection/retrieval procedure.

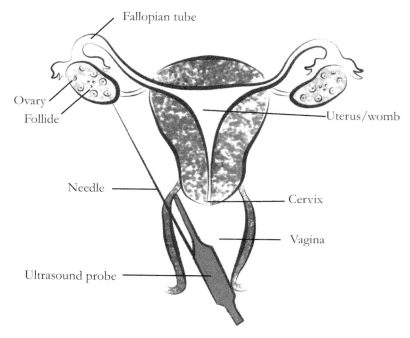

Fallopian tube

Ovary

Follide

Uterus/womb

Needle

Cervix

Vagina

Ultrasound probe

Egg Donor – ED

This explanation is more about the woman who donates her eggs rather than the woman who uses donor eggs to have a baby. See 'Donor Egg" for further information about receiving a donated egg.

An egg donor is a woman who donates some of her eggs to be used by another woman who can't use her own eggs in order to get pregnant. She may decide to donate her eggs to help someone she knows, like a family member or a friend, or she does it for altruistic reasons.

In some countries, only her expenses are paid but in other countries a donor can be paid a lot of money depending on their education, family background, physical characteristics etc.

In some countries the egg donor is anonymous but in others, like the UK, any children born as a result of your donation can, when they reach 18 years old, find out some information about you, such as your name and last known address.

If a woman decides to donate her eggs she must fulfil certain criteria:

- be between certain ages, generally between 18 and 35 years old
- be free of any serious diseases or medical conditions that could affect the mother or baby
- must not have any inheritable diseases in her family.

Her ovarian reserve, that is how many egg cells she has left in her ovaries, may also be tested and her body mass index (BMI) may be taken into consideration.

How much information the recipient receives about the donor varies from country to country – in some countries they will know very little, only such things as age, hair colour, eye colour, job and hobbies, whereas in other countries, they will see the donor's photo, know about their education and qualifications, personal achievements and family history.

The donor will go through an IVF cycle, taking the medication, having the blood tests and scans, up to the point of the egg collection/retrieval, EC/ER. The donor has no legal rights or responsibilities over any children born from their donation. By law in the UK a donor must be offered counselling and this is strongly recommended so that they can think about all the implications of their decision and how it could affect their own future family. To find out more about egg donation in the country you live in, contact the fertility authority body or visit their website.

Egg Freezing/Cryopreservation

Also known as 'vitrification', this is the method by which eggs are frozen. Egg freezing was originally used for women who were about to have treatment that would affect the quality of their eggs, such as cancer treatment, or women who had medical conditions that affected their fertility. Nowadays, it is also commonly used by women who are in their 20s or 30s who would like to have a biological baby in the future, when they have either met a partner and/or when they are older but their egg quality will not be so good. This is known as 'elective egg freezing'. It may also be used if you are undergoing a sex change operation.

You will have to undergo an IVF cycle which means injecting or sniffing hormonal medication in order to stimulate your ovaries to produce a large number of mature eggs. From the start of the procedure to the end can take between two and three weeks. Your eggs will be collected or retrieved under sedation or general anaesthetic – see 'Egg Collection/Retrieval' for more information. You may have to do more than one IVF cycle in order to achieve a large number of eggs because it's likely that not all your eggs will survive the freezing or the thawing. There have been instances where no eggs have survived.

Instead of your eggs being fertilised with sperm, they are dehydrated and the fluid replaced with a solution called cryoprotectant, which is like antifreeze, preventing ice crystals from forming; these could damage your eggs when they are thawed in the future. Your eggs are then frozen and stored in tanks of liquid nitrogen at a temperature of -196°C. When you want to use your eggs in the future to start your family, your eggs will be thawed and those that have survived and are normal will be fertilised with either your partner's sperm or a donor's sperm, usually using ICSI.

Obviously, the cost of IVF and freezing your eggs varies from country to country, and there is also the yearly cost of storage. If you are considering freezing your eggs, do your research and go to a clinic that is experienced and ask to see their most recent success rates for women in your age group.

In the UK you can store your eggs for up to ten years; in exceptional circumstances, up to 55 years. In other countries this will vary; for example, in Southern California in the United States, you can freeze your eggs for as long as you need to.

Egg Quality

Currently there is no egg quality test that can be carried out on your eggs. The best indication that is used for your egg quality is your age. Our eggs start to develop when we ourselves are developing in our mother's womb, and they are very fragile and susceptible to all sorts of damage, such as:

- fever
- infection
- stress
- free radicals.

Over the years, this damage builds up and causes chromosomal abnormalities in your eggs, so when you are in your 20s, there has been less time for your eggs to be exposed to damage so they will be a better quality than your eggs when you are in your late 30s for example. Even in your 20s some of your eggs will have chromosomal abnormalities. Once an egg is damaged, it cannot be healed. Even if you have led a healthy lifestyle and haven't smoked or drunk copious amounts of alcohol every weekend, your egg quality will deteriorate over time. We all probably know of a woman who possibly had smoked and almost definitely drunk alcohol previously and was in her 40s when she got pregnant naturally, and her baby was born healthily (thankfully) – with nature there is sometimes no rhyme or reason. Consider asking your mother at what age she had her menopause or how old she was when she had you or your younger sibling(s) as genetics plays a part.

There is no denying that your egg quality is directly related to the chances of you getting pregnant either naturally or with fertility treatment. Once a month (if you have regular menstrual cycles), one egg matures when ovulation occurs, and that one egg is the one chance for you to get pregnant in that month. It may be normal or it may not, and if it isn't, even if it is fertilised, there is a higher chance that you will miscarry. Even if you do IVF with your own eggs and you are older, how successful you are is about the same as trying to get pregnant naturally.

The average percentage of embryos (fertilised eggs) that are genetically normal when you are:

- 30 years of age is approximately 70%
- 38 years of age is approximately 50%
- 40 years of age is approximately 40%
- 43 years of age is approximately 10%.

Although it is believed that you cannot improve your egg quality or heal damaged eggs, you can look after the quality of your healthy eggs by thinking about your lifestyle in the following ways (I'm not guaranteeing that you will get pregnant but you have to eat and look after yourself so why not do it for your fertility health?):

1. Ensure your hormones are balanced correctly by eating essential fatty acids found in tuna, salmon, avocado and coconut oil. Cut down on Omega-6 foods such as sunflower oil, canola oil and baked dairy goods. Consider mediation to reduce stress. Get more vitamin D into your body – see 'Vitamin D' for more information. Do some

exercise such as the housework and walking the dog. Get 7-10 hours of sleep – see 'Sleep' for more information

2. Protect your eggs and reproductive organs (and your partner's sperm and his organs) from free radical damage. If you drink, smoke and/or take drugs, stopping is best but at least cut down. If your diet consists of processed foods, change it so that your diet includes lots of foods rich in antioxidants, such as bright coloured fruits and vegetables.

3. Nourish your eggs' development and health by eating proteins, such as fish, chicken, broccoli, peas and lentils, but don't go overboard as too much protein can negatively affect fertility. Also ensure you get enough Vitamin D3. Always seek medical advice regard supplements.

4. Improve the blood flow to your reproductive organs.

5. Reduce your (and your partner's) exposure to chemicals such as bisphenol A (BPA) and perfluorooctanoic acid (PFOA). Most harmful chemicals are found in household products such as plastic containers, plastic water drinking bottles and plastic food wrap.

6. Vitamin B8 is important for all cells, and especially for the development of your follicles, blastocyst development and maintaining blood sugar balance. It has been found in the follicle fluid of good quality eggs. It is found in fruits, especially cantaloupe melon and grapefruit, fresh vegetables (these are better than frozen or canned), beans and grains, particularly oats and bran, and nuts, especially almond and walnuts. Please seek medical advice regard supplements.

7. Manage your stress as chronic stress can affect ovulation and cause problems with fertilisation and implantation. Even 20 minutes a day doing something where you slow down, like yoga, meditation and breathing, will have a benefit.

The below is not to scale and is an artistic impression of your egg.

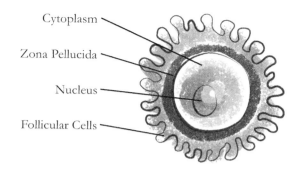

Cytoplasm

Zona Pellucida

Nucleus

Follicular Cells

Egg Retrieval – ER

See 'Egg Collection' for more information.

Egg Sharing

This is what you can do if you are doing an IVF cycle. If applicable to your fertility clinic, they give you a discount on the cost of your cycle if you give some of your eggs to another woman or couple. In order to egg share, you will need to produce enough eggs during the cycle for yourself and the other woman, known as the 'recipient', who will receive an equal share of your eggs. In order to egg share, you do need to fulfil certain criteria, similar to a woman who is an egg donor, with the addition that your clinic may also check your ovarian reserve. See 'Egg Donor' for more information.

In the UK it is not possible for you or the recipient to meet, but you can set certain conditions as to how your eggs are used, providing there is no discrimination against people with protected characteristics under the Equality Act 2010.

This is a huge decision to make as in effect you are becoming an egg donor, and your clinic should not put any pressure on you. You must consider the emotional side of egg sharing – how will you feel if the recipient has a baby and you don't and in the future the child tries to get in contact with you? In the UK, the law is that children born following egg donation can request the name and last known address of the donor when they turn 18. All clinics in the UK by law must offer you implications counselling or you can seek this out yourself.

Ejaculation

This is when semen, a fluid that usually contains sperm, is pumped out of the penis with rhythmic contractions.

Elective Egg Freezing

See 'Egg Freezing' for more information.

Elective Single Embryo Transfer – eSET

This is when a single embryo is selected from a number of embryos and is transferred back to your womb during your ART cycle, such as IVF. All other suitable embryos are then frozen. The reason for eSET rather than transferring more than one embryo is to reduce multiple births and the risks to you and your babies. In some clinics in some countries it is still quite common for more than one embryo to be transferred.

Even in clinics who practise eSET, your doctor may decide that with your history and your circumstances, transferring more than one embryo may give you a better chance of having a baby. It is very important that you discuss your embryo transfer with your doctor and consider the future of having twins or triplets or more.

Electro Stim Acupuncture or Electroacupuncture

This is acupuncture with needles with a slight electrical current or pulse. It gives the acupuncturist more control over the amount of stimulation provided to acupuncture points. See 'Acupuncture' for more information.

Embryo – Emby/Embaby

This develops from a sperm fertilising an egg. Between fertilisation and Day 4 the correct name is a 'zygote' but nobody involved in fertility treatments uses this term, preferring the term 'embryo'. It is technically an 'embryo' from the fourth day after fertilisation to the end of the eighth week of pregnancy.

Please note: the illustration below is not to scale nor accurate with regard to embryo grading; it is more to give you a bit of an idea of what a developing embryo from Day 2 to Day 5 looks like.

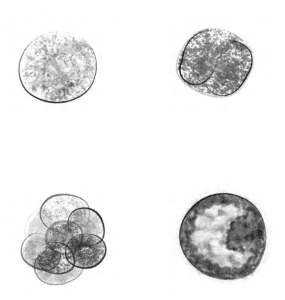

Embryo Adoption

This is when a woman or a couple (recipient/s) who cannot get pregnant using their own embryo 'adopt' an embryo from another woman (donor) in the hope of getting pregnant. The recipient and donor may know each and make the arrangement themselves, or it may be anonymous via a fertility clinic. The donor will have gone through an IVF procedure to produce eggs and the eggs will have been fertilised by her partner's sperm or donor sperm. You, as the recipient, may receive a fresh embryo or a frozen embryo and the embryo transfer is the same procedure as an egg transfer, and will be carried out at an optimum time in your menstrual cycle.

There may be legal aspects in some countries, just as when a child is adopted.

As with a donor egg or donor sperm, the baby born following embryo adoption is absolutely your baby, and don't let anyone tell you differently, as you have carried the baby in your womb exactly as you would if the baby had been made from your egg and your partner's sperm (or from a sperm donor). You have felt the baby move, you have fed the baby and protected it and the baby has heard your, and your partner's/family's/friends' voices. From a legal perspective, you have given birth to the baby and you are their legal mother and, if you are married or are in a civil partnership, your husband/partner will be the legal father.

Embryo Cryopreservation/Freezing – EC

During ART such as IVF, it is hoped that a number of eggs are collected and fertilised. As only one or two embryos are transferred back into your womb, it is possible that you have embryos left over. These embryos will be assessed for quality and, if they are at the correct stage of their development on the day of transfer, a decision will be made about whether they are suitable for cryopreservation/freezing – either to be used in a future cycle if this cycle isn't successful, or for a sibling if this cycle is successful. Suitable embryos are the ones most likely to survive the freezing process and the thawing process if used in a future cycle.

Embryos are frozen using an ultra-rapid freezing method called 'vitrification', the same as freezing eggs. You will have this process explained to you at your clinic because you have to sign a consent form. In the UK, the standard storage time that frozen embryos can be kept is 10 years (though it can be up to 55 years) and it varies from country to country where embryo freezing is allowed. Most fertility clinics freeze embryos and eggs but ask before you start treatment. This also is an important question if you are doing treatment in a country where you don't live. There will be a fee to pay for the freezing and the future storage.

Embryo Donation

This is when another couple or a woman donate her/their embryo/s to another woman or couple who cannot get pregnant with her own eggs or their own embryo. Those who donate embryos usually do so when they have had their babies and completed their family and who want to help someone else become a parent. They may do it anonymously or they may be related to the woman/couple who will receive the embryo.

See 'Embryo Adoption' for more information.

Embryoglue

This is the brand name of a product used in ART such as IVF that you may see on forums/support groups etc. As with many products used in fertility treatments, some experts believe the product is required and others do not believe it is necessary, so always do your research and ask questions.

Some clinics may use this product as part of your treatment so there will be no extra charge for it; other clinics may charge if you want to use the product during your treatment.

Please note: I am not suggesting you use this product and I have no relationship with the company that produces it, I have simply included it in this book because it is mentioned on forums and your clinic may mention it during your appointment.

Embryo Grading

This is another nerve-wracking part of IVF and ICSI etc that you have no choice but to go through. Once your eggs have been fertilised in the laboratory, the embryologist checks them on a regular basis and during their development they are 'graded'. The process is subjective and it will differ from clinic to clinic, so comparing your embryo's grades to someone else's doesn't help at all, and embryos that have been transferred and did not receive a good grade have gone on to implant and create a baby. Similarly, embryos with fantastic grades have sadly ended in a negative pregnancy test or a miscarriage.

Your embryos are first given a grade two days after your egg collection, i.e. Day 2. They can also be graded on Days 3, 5 and 6 but not usually on Day 4. Day 2 and 3 embryos are given a grade of 4, 3, 2, or 1; 4 being the highest or the best and 1 being the poorest quality.

A Day 2 embryo is called a 'cleavage stage embryo' and will be between two and four cells. The embryologist grades on how even the cells are and if there is any fragmentation – see 'Fragmentation' for more information. An embryo with more even cells and very little fragmentation will receive a better grade and will be classed as a better-quality embryo.

A Day 3 embryo is also called a 'cleavage stage embryo' and will be between 6 and 8 cells. They are graded the same way as a Day 2 embryo.

Once your embryo reaches the blastocyst stage, so Day 5, if it has not been transferred already, it is graded slightly differently, because a blastocyst now contains two distinct types of cells: one type forms the baby and the other type the placenta. Each cell type is given a grade, so a blastocyst is graded with a number and two letters, for example 4AA. The baby-making cells should be visible under a microscope and a blastocyst with a large group of these cells will receive a higher grade than one with a smaller group of cells (A being the highest, then B then C). The placenta-making cells should be long and flat and be continuous; if there are any holes or large cells this group of cells will get a lower grade. The number refers to the degree that the embryo has expanded and its progress towards hatching out of its zona pellucinda, a bit like an eggshell, and is on a scale of 1-6. The ideal Day 5 blastocyst would score 4AA which would mean it has expanded as expected and both cell types are excellent.

If it scores a number 5 it means it has started to hatch and a number 6 indicates it has completely hatched.

Please note: the illustration below is not to scale nor accurate with regard to embryo grading; it is more to give you a bit of an idea of what a developing embryo from Day 2 to Day 5 looks like.

6-18 hours after
fertilisation

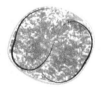

Day 2: cleaved
embryo

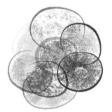

Day 3: 8 cell
embryo

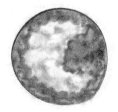

Day 5-6: blastocyst

Embryologist

This is a scientist not a medical doctor and s/he looks after the eggs, sperm, embryos and blastocysts in the laboratory at the clinic. They spend most of their time in the laboratory preparing the eggs and sperm, checking on the embryos/blastocysts and keeping meticulous records. In some clinics the embryologist will speak to you about your embryos, either in person or on the phone, and in other clinics you may never speak to them as the information is passed onto you via another member of the team. You may see them at the clinic as they are usually wearing blue trousers and top, like doctors' wear in theatres in hospitals, or a white lab coat and often have a disposable hat covering their hair. When they are in the laboratory they are usually wearing masks.

Below is an artistic impression of an embryologist viewing a Day 2 embryo.

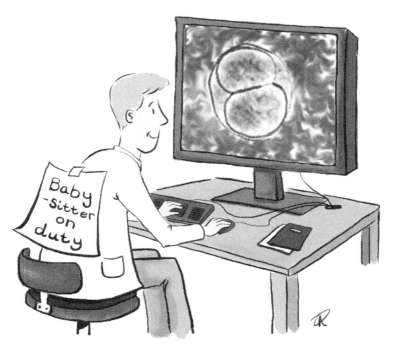

Embryo Monitoring

See 'Time Lapse Monitoring' for more information.

Embryo Sharing

See 'Embryo Donation' and 'Embryo Adoption'.

Embryo Squishiness

This is something you may read about as it is quite a new development in ART such as IVF. Some embryos apparently are squishier than others, and scientists believe that an embryo with the correct amount of squishiness has a better chance of implanting and going on to become a baby. Currently it is unknown why this correct amount of squishiness makes a difference but it is thought to have something to do with the DNA.

Embryo Toxicity Assay – ETA and Embryo Toxicity Factor – ETF

This is a test that you might consider if you have had recurrent miscarriages, unexplained infertility and recurrent IVF cycle failures.

It is a blood test that is done to find out if your body is producing a substance called 'embryonic toxic factor' or ETF; this is toxic to your embryo and could cause miscarriages or implantation failures. ETF is produced by the white blood cells in your immune system (the system in your body that fights infections, foreign bodies etc) during a normal pregnancy. If your white blood cells produce more ETF than they should, your immune system may attack your embryo as it thinks it is a foreign body, which results in implantation failure naturally or following IVF, and/or a miscarriage.

Embryo Transfer – ET

This is the moment you have been waiting for. All your hard work is about to pay off. You'll likely feel nervous, excited, scared, positive and negative in equal measures and all at once, but you'll be used to this by now. These feelings are totally normal and felt by everyone. ET usually occurs on Day 2 (i.e. two days after egg collection/retrieval or EC/ER, EC being Day 0), or Day 3 or Day 5. On forums, when in the Two-Week Wait, you may see '3dp2dt' which means the woman is '3 days post a Day 2 embryo transfer'. Whether you are having an embryo or a blastocyst transferred back into your womb, generally everyone calls it 'ET'. Your embryo will be transferred to the best possible home: your womb.

Your ET is a much simpler procedure than your EC/ER. Your clinic will arrange the time for you to go in, and it is very similar to having a smear/pap smear – you are awake, you lie on your back with your legs in stirrups and a speculum is inserted into your vagina…. you get the idea.

Just before the transfer an amazing event takes place – most clinics show you (and your partner) on a monitor your actual embryo/s: your future child/ren. How amazing is that! You may even get given a photo or emailed the photo of your embryo/s. This is usually a really emotional time and don't be surprised if you have tears in your eyes and a lump in your throat as you are looking at your future baby; what an absolute privilege. One small bonus and a positive side of having had to do ART.

Some clinics do the ET in the operating theatre so you will probably put on a gown; other clinics do it in a side room. Your partner/ friend may be allowed to go with you; again, all clinics are different so you may want to check beforehand. Once you are ready, a thin plastic tube called a catheter, which contains your embryo in the culture that has been nourishing it, is passed through your cervix and into your womb. Some clinics use an ultrasound scan to guide them and others don't believe it helps. You may have had what is called a 'trial transfer' during a previous appointment where the doctor/nurse ensures the catheter goes through your cervix with no problems, or they may do it before your actual transfer. Once the transfer has taken place, the catheter is checked under a microscope by the embryologist to ensure it is empty, which indicates the transfer was successful.

Sheila says: There aren't many things that are nice about doing IVF etc but I always try and see a positive in everything and I always felt, at ET, that for once, we are so much luckier that those women who conceive naturally – they don't get this absolutely amazing experience of meeting their future child at two, three or five days after fertilisation. We do and when you finally hold your baby in your arms and you think back to seeing them as an embryo, wow! you realise again that they are little miracles. Oh, and by the way, this feeling never goes away.

Emotional Freedom Technique – EFT

Also called 'tapping'. This is a set of techniques which uses the body's energy meridian points by tapping on them with your fingertips. It is similar to acupuncture but without the needles.

A very simple explanation is that you focus on the negative emotion at hand: it could be a fear or anxiety, a bad memory, or anything that's bothering you. While maintaining your mental focus on your emotion, tap with your fingertips five to seven times each on 12 of the body's meridian points. Tapping on these meridian points – while concentrating on and talking through the negative emotion – accesses your body's energy, restoring it to a balanced state.

Scepticism surrounds whether it works or not; you are either a believer or not. Recent research has shown that the brain's stress and fear response – which is controlled by a part of your brain called the amygdala – could be lessened by stimulating the meridian points. EFT is being used by women who are struggling to get pregnant.

Empty Follicle Syndrome – EFS

This is fortunately a very uncommon complication in ART, such as IVF. It is frustrating for the team who are looking after you but devastating if you experience it. It means that at egg collection/retrieval (EC/ER) no eggs are collected from your follicles, despite ultrasound and oestradiol measurements indicating that you have many follicles.

It is believed to be down to human error, for example mistiming of administering the trigger shot, or your eggs are immature and are very tightly stuck to the follicle wall so won't come unstuck.

Endometrial Biopsy – EB/EMB

This is when a sample of your endometrium/womb lining is taken for laboratory analysis.

The reasons for it being carried out are if you have irregular, heavy, or prolonged bleeding or if an ultrasound scan shows a thickened uterine lining. When it is being carried out for investigations into infertility, it is to check the lining of your womb to determine if it is being prepared by your hormones, namely oestrogen, adequately for a fertilised egg to implant.

It's a minor procedure taking about 10 minutes and is similar to a smear/pap smear in how it is carried out; you lie down with your legs in stirrups and once the doctor has cleaned your vagina and cervix with a cold solution, they insert a speculum into your vagina; this part can be uncomfortable (and embarrassing). The doctor then passes a thin, flexible tube through into your womb where they gently move it around to obtain a small sample of your endometrial lining. The sample of tissue is placed in a solution and sent for analysis. It can be uncomfortable during the procedure, and you may have some light spotting or bleeding afterwards so you may want to wear a sanitary pad (or similar) but not tampons, and if you have any cramping after take a pain killer. Don't have sex for several days to reduce the possibility of infection.

See 'Endometrium' for more information. It is also the same procedure for the endometrial receptivity array test – see below for more information.

Endometrial Receptivity Array Test – ERA

This is a relatively new diagnostic technique sometimes used in ART such as IVF. It is a genetic test that evaluates whether your endometrial lining has properly developed and is ready for an embryo to implant, otherwise known as your 'implantation window.' This is only a small window as it usually occurs around days 19-21 of your menstrual cycle, and for about 80% of us, our implantation window occurs in this time frame. However, for approximately 20% of us, we have a unique window that is outside of the usual implantation window. Therefore, transferring an embryo back to your womb when it is not ready may result in implantation failure. It may be recommended if you have had recurrent implantation failures, i.e. two or more unsuccessful transfers.

In order to test the endometrial lining, a procedure called an endometrial biopsy is carried out as an outpatient without anaesthetic. See 'Endometrial Biopsy' (above) for more information.

The sample that is collected is then tested and classified as 'receptive' or 'non-receptive'. Doing this procedure now enables a clinic to personalise your embryo transfer (pET). The below is not to scale and is an artistic impression of your reproductive system.

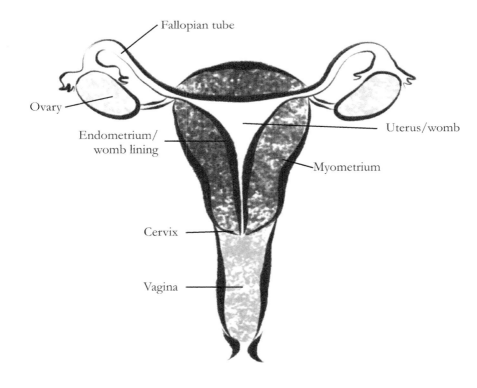

Endometrial Scratch

Also called 'womb scratching', this is a relatively new procedure that may be carried out during your ART cycle such as IVF. The endometrium is a layer of tissue lining the inside of your uterus or womb.

When the embryo arrives in your womb after its journey down your Fallopian tube, it attaches or implants itself into the endometrium and will (hopefully) remain there for the next nine months. When the embryo is transferred to your womb during IVF or any other ART cycle, it will hopefully implant successfully and also remain there for the next nine months. It is thought by some experts that by scratching the endometrium an inflammatory response occurs similar to when you have a scratch on another part of your body, and when the wound heals, the healing response creates a new lining that may be more receptive to an embryo to implant and remain there.

The procedure is carried out as an outpatient without anaesthetic and only takes a couple of minutes. Like most procedures that involve your womb, it is similar to a pap/smear; you lie down with your legs in stirrups and once the doctor has cleaned your vagina and cervix with a cold solution, they insert a speculum into your vagina; this part can be uncomfortable (and embarrassing). A thin, flexible plastic tube is then inserted through your cervix into your womb where it is moved around in order to scratch/injure the lining. It can cause discomfort and pain and rare complications are infection and uterine perforation. It is carried out a week or so prior to the start of an ART cycle or frozen embryo transfer (FET).

This procedure maybe suggested to you if you have had multiple unsuccessful ART cycles despite transferring good quality embryos/blastocysts. The evidence as to whether having an endometrial scratch will increase your chances of having a baby is currently inconclusive mainly because trials that have been carried out are too small.

Endometriosis – Endo

This is a common, long-term condition caused by tissue that mimics the lining of your womb/uterus called your 'endometrium', and this tissue is found in other parts of your body, such as your:

- Fallopian tubes
- ovaries
- stomach, and
- in or around your bladder and bowel.

The cause is unknown but it may be hereditary or be due to something called 'metaplasia', which is when cells in your body change into a different kind of cell following an inflammation. Symptoms vary a lot and some women are badly affected whilst others less so. Symptoms include the following:

- period pain not relieved by painkillers
- heavy periods where you need to wear extra pads or change your tampon frequently
- pelvic pain either around the time of your period or the pain is constant
- pain during and after sex
- discomfort or pain when you pee or poo
- blood in your poo or bleeding from your bottom
- feeling constantly tired.

For some, the symptoms are so bad it stops them from leading a normal life and can lead to depression. As it is quite a difficult condition to diagnose, a laparoscopy may be required. Treatment varies but can include anti-inflammatory painkillers such as ibuprofen, hormone medicines and contraceptives or surgery.

The main complication is that it can cause problems when trying to get pregnant. If you have severe endometriosis it can cause scarring/adhesions, your Fallopian tubes can become damaged and/or blocked and your ovaries can contain cysts. However, many women with even severe endometriosis do get pregnant without needing fertility treatment.

Endometrium

Also called the womb lining, as it is the tissue that lines the cavity of your womb/uterus. Your womb is an upside-down, pear-shaped, hollow reproductive organ that is in your pelvic area. At the beginning of your menstrual cycle your ovaries produce a hormone called oestrogen/estrogen which is responsible for creating a nice thick blood-rich endometrium, ready to accept a fertilised egg. Your endometrium grows roughly 1-2 mm every day and a healthy uterine lining is 8-13 mm thick (this figure varies from clinic to clinic). If it is thinner than this, a fertilised egg is unlikely to implant. If your oestrogen/estrogen levels are not as they should be your endometrium will not thicken.

Around the middle of your cycle (just after ovulation), your ovaries start producing a hormone called progesterone which prepares the innermost layer of the endometrium to support the embryo should it implant. If pregnancy occurs, the developing placenta begins to secrete hCG (human chorionic gonadotropin) also known as the 'pregnancy hormone', which tells the corpus luteum (what was previously the follicle the egg was in), to carry on producing progesterone which ensures the endometrium keeps nourishing the embryo. If pregnancy doesn't happen, the corpus luteum starts to break down, which causes the progesterone levels to drop dramatically and this innermost layer is shed as your menstrual period.

You can see how it is really important that the balance of all these hormones has to be absolutely perfect if you are going to get pregnant naturally. When you are doing fertility treatment such as IVF, the hormone levels are unlikely to be the same as the levels found during a normal menstrual cycle, and this is maybe why some fertility clinics often suggest that you freeze your embryos and then, a couple of months later, have a defrosted embryo transferred to your womb during your natural menstrual cycle.

However, it is not only hormones that ensure the endometrium is ready to receive and nourish an embryo and therefore help you to become pregnant. It must also be smooth and not have any abnormalities such as fibroids, polyps, endometriosis, scar tissue, adhesions or adenomyosis (when the endometrium breaks through the muscle wall of your womb).

It must also have a good blood flow or it won't thicken. Your blood flow may not be adequate if you:

- have a sedentary lifestyle with little exercise
- have fibroids that are pressing on blood vessels
- have chronic stress which can constrict (squeeze) blood vessels that carry blood to your womb.

Around the time of ovulation your womb contracts more frequently, possibly to help sperm move from the cervix up to your Fallopian tubes to reach and fertilise the egg. It usually stops contracting five to six days later, about the time when implantation occurs due to the production of progesterone. If you are doing IVF or other fertility treatment, it isn't unusual for you to experience some cramping around the time you have your embryo/s transferred due to all the prodding and poking that has gone on around your ovaries and womb.

A recent theory that is still being researched is the belief that a viral infection of the endometrium may be the cause of recurrent miscarriage and unexplained infertility. The virus is believed to be part of the herpes simplex family, the same virus that causes chicken pox and cold sores. Even after the initial infection has gone, the virus remains dormant in your body.

The below is not to scale and is an artistic impression of your reproductive system.

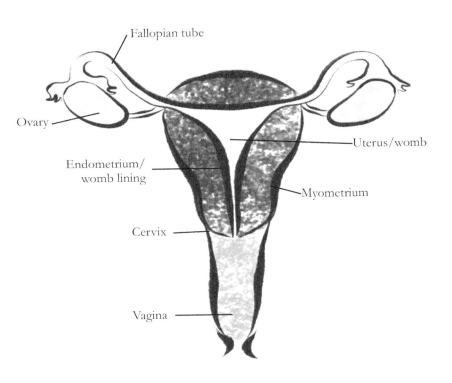

Epididymitis

This is an inflammation of the epididymis, which is a tube that stores and carries sperm at the back of each testicle/testis. It can affect men of all ages but more often between the age of 14 and 35 years old. It is usually caused by a bacterial infection or a sexually transmitted disease (STD), such as chlamydia or gonorrhoea. Symptoms include

- pain in the pelvic area
- pain and tenderness in the testicles
- pain during intercourse and ejaculation
- passing pee frequently.

It can be acute, lasting less than six weeks; or chronic, lasting longer than six weeks. It can cause infertility:

- by the epididymis tube becoming blocked from scar tissue due to an infection or repeated infections
- by the testicles themselves become damaged, resulting in no sperm being produced
- due to a low sperm count because the functionality of the scrotum (which stores sperm) is affected
- by the man having anti-sperm antibodies – see 'Anti-sperm Antibodies' for more information.

Treatment will depend very much on the cause.

The below is not to scale and is an artistic impression of the male reproductive system.

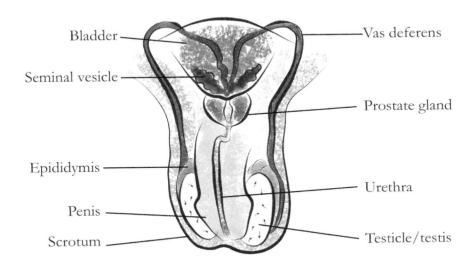

Bladder

Vas deferens

Seminal vesicle

Prostate gland

Epididymis

Urethra

Penis

Scrotum

Testicle/testis

Epigenetics

If you use donor eggs to have your baby, your body is still influencing your baby's genes by passing on your own genetic material through your endometrial fluid. Your baby will look very different to the baby that the donor would have given birth to had she got pregnant with the egg she donated to you. Many parents of donor egg-conceived babies have said how their baby looks like its mummy or another member of the mother's family.

Your body contains trillions of cells and almost all of them contain the instructions that make you, you. These instructions are your DNA. The DNA is organised into chromosomes – we have 23 pairs of chromosomes, so 46 in total. Chromosomes are organised into genes and each person has the same set of genes, some 20,000 in all. We all have a gene for hair colour, a gene for whether our hair is curly or straight, whether our eye colour is blue, brown or hazel and so on. But we do have different versions of these genes and it's these versions that dictate what colour our hair is, or our eyes are, or whether our hair is curly or not.

Epigenetics instructs the DNA what to do and it is influenced by external factors:

- the environment the developing baby lives in, i.e. your womb
- the environment you live in
- the food you eat that nourishes your baby
- your behaviour
- what illnesses and diseases you have.

This is why your baby that started from a donor's egg is absolutely and totally your child.

Epilepsy

Women, and men, with epilepsy may have a slightly higher risk of reduced fertility than someone who doesn't have epilepsy. If you have epilepsy your medication will affect the pituitary gland, which could cause ovulation problems. Your menstrual cycle may be affected by your epilepsy, your epilepsy medication, the number of seizures you have and your age. Studies indicate that if you have epilepsy and are taking a certain medication, you are more likely to be affected by PCOS, though any woman can be affected with PCOS. If you are concerned that you may have PCOS, you must not stop taking your medication but must speak to your doctor about your concerns.

In men, the effects of certain anti-epileptic drugs were studied and abnormal sperm morphology and motility were often seen.

Estradiol/Oestradiol – E2

See 'Oestradiol/ Oestrogen/Oestriol' for more information.

European Society of Human Reproduction and Embryology – ESHRE

The main aim of this society is to promote interest in and understanding of reproductive biology and medicine. It promotes improvements in clinical practice through organising teaching and training activities, and providing guidance to improve safety and quality in procedures. Every year ESHRE organises a meeting in a European country and people from around the world attend.

Evacuation of Retained Products of Conception – ERPC

A horrible term that should be changed. See 'Dilation & Evacuation' for more information.

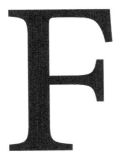

FACTOR V LEIDEN THROMBOPHILIA

to

FROZEN EMBRYO TRANSFER

The hypothalamus (a gland in your brain) is approximately the size of a pea.

Factor V Leiden Thrombophilia

This is a genetic disorder that means you have more of a tendency than others to form abnormal blood clots that can block your blood vessels, and you may be more likely to develop blood clots during pregnancy or when taking the hormone oestrogen/estrogen.

It is believed by some fertility experts that if you have the Factor V Leiden mutation* it means you may have an increased risk of recurrent miscarriages after 10 weeks, possibly due to tiny blood clots blocking the flow of nutrients to the placenta.

Treatment is with blood-thinning medication.

*Mutation simply means the structure of the gene has been changed.

Fallopian Tubes

These are a pair of long, narrow tubes about 10 cm long that connect your ovaries to your womb. When you ovulate, an egg travels down one of your Fallopian tubes to your womb. The egg may be fertilised by sperm in the tube. One or both tubes can become blocked or damaged by:

- pelvic infections
- surgery
- endometriosis
- fibroids
- scar tissue.

Diagnosis of blocked Fallopian tube(s) is confirmed by a hysterosalpingography – see 'Blocked Fallopian Tubes' for more information. If one tube is blocked this shouldn't be a cause of infertility providing you are ovulating from both ovaries. However, if both your tubes are blocked this can be a cause of infertility.

The below is not to scale and is an artistic impression of your reproductive system.

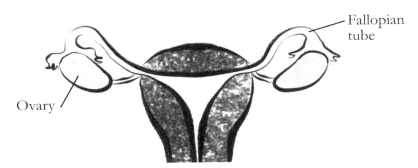

Fertile Window

The number of days in your menstrual cycle when you are at your most fertile. See 'Fertility Monitor' and 'Follicular Phase' for more information.

Fertilisation

This is when a sperm enters an egg and the DNA from the sperm combines with the DNA from the egg in order to create a new life. This happens naturally in the Fallopian tube and then the fertilised egg travels to your womb where it hopefully embeds in your womb lining. During ART such as IVF, it occurs in the fertility clinic's laboratory with the help of an embryologist. But it is still a miracle.

The below is not to scale and is an artistic impression of fertilisation.

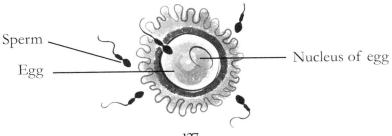

Fertility Blend

This is a brand of fertility supplements for women and men that you may see mentioned on forums, hence including it here. I do not endorse this product nor do I have any association with the company.

Fertility Cleanse

This is something you may want to do before you get pregnant or before you start fertility treatment. Cleansing the body has been around for thousands of years and was used by Egyptians, Japanese and Native Americans. It is believed fertility cleansing specifically supports your body in preparation for getting pregnant by cleansing your womb and liver.

If you decide to do a fertility cleanse be sure to seek the advice of a specialist in this area.

Fertility Cliff

The is the term often used by doctors and the press, and it is referring to the belief that when you reach a certain age – around 35 – your chances of getting pregnant and having a baby steeply drop.

Fertility Coach

This is someone who supports and guides you, and possibly your partner, on your fertility journey. They will help you to achieve your fertility goals, such as creating healthy lifestyle habits in order to increase your chances of conceiving. They will help you to keep moving forwards even when you think you are stuck. They help you to create an environment that promotes not only a fertile body but also a fertile mind and spirit. Often a fertility coach also practices nutrition, hypnotherapy, acupuncture and mindfulness, to name a few.

Fertility Counsellor

This is someone who will have trained as a counsellor and specialises in counselling people who are finding it challenging to get pregnant. Counselling is where two people meet privately and regularly with the aim of restoring emotional well-being for you, the client. It provides you with a safe place to be yourself and to say what you truly feel without the fear of judgement, criticism or unwanted advice. When there is something in your life that is getting you down, counselling can help you to understand your emotions more clearly.

Sheila says: I would absolutely recommend counselling or coaching if you are having fertility treatment. You might think you are coping and it isn't necessary but often the emotional cost of fertility treatment doesn't show itself until later, especially if you have experienced a number of failed cycles of treatment. According to the HFEA in the UK, if you are doing IVF, ICSI or any other variations of IVF, you should legally be offered counselling by your clinic prior to any treatment starting, and the counsellor should be attached to the clinic (though if you prefer otherwise, they should provide you with a list of suitable counsellors). The length of time you see a counsellor for, if you choose to, is up to you and you can see them on your own or with your partner (if you are doing treatment with a partner). This advice may be different in other countries.

Fertility Europe

A European network of various organisations who are dedicated to infertility. Their aim is to raise infertility awareness through communication, education, advocacy and partnerships, and also to share best practices between those who work with infertility patients. In 2016 they organised the first European Fertility Week (EFW); this is now an annual event occurring the first week in November.

Fertility Massage

Also known as 'sacral abdominal massage', fertility massage aims to bring balance and harmony to the reproductive, digestive and sacral areas (the bottom of your spine). Massage helps to increase blood flow to the uterus and ovaries and reconnects you to your body, and especially to your womb. If you want to consider fertility massage, you do need to see a therapist who has been trained in fertility massage and not a general 'spa-type' therapist.

Fertility Monitor – FM

This is an electronic device that helps you to understand your fertility. It provides you with information as to when is the best time that you will conceive:

- the couple of days before you ovulate

- when you ovulate

- when is the best time to have sex.

This is often referred to as your 'fertile window'. A monitor works by analysing hormonal changes in either urine, saliva or cervical mucus, or changes in your body temperature or a combination. There are a number of different ones on the market to choose from, so do your research as some are better than others if, for example, you have PCOS. Some also have apps.

Fertility MOT

This is a consultation with a fertility expert to discuss the results from two tests, the 'anti-Müllerian hormone' (AMH) and antral follicle count (AFC), as well as reviewing your medical history, especially your gynaecological and your fertility.

Some experts believe that the Fertility MOT isn't a good idea – if your results come back 'normal' this does not mean that you will be able to get pregnant in the future, and an 'abnormal' result doesn't mean that you won't be able to get pregnant in the future.

See 'Anti-Müllerian Hormone' and 'Antral Follicle Count' for more information.

Fertility Mucus – FM

See 'Cervical Mucus' for more information.

Fertility Network – FN UK

Before 2017 this was known as Infertility Network UK or IN UK. It is the main UK charity that helps anyone who has ever experienced fertility problems. They provide:

- free and impartial support

- information

- advice

- understanding, as a majority of the people who work there have experienced fertility challenges.

They campaign for equal access to NHS treatment and work with the media to raise public awareness on all aspects of fertility issues. They are associated with the UK Fertility Shows in London and Manchester and organise the annual Fertility Awareness Week during the first week of November.

Fertility Nurse

This is a qualified nurse who has specialised in fertility and works as part of the multi-professional team at the fertility clinic, either carrying out or assisting with your fertility investigations and treatment. You generally speak to the fertility nurse during fertility treatments more than other members of the team.

Fibroids

These are very common, non-cancerous growths that are found in or around your womb. They are made up of muscle and fibrous tissue and vary in size. Their cause is unknown but it's thought their development is connected to hormones, namely oestrogen/ estrogen and progesterone. They can cause infertility by:

- blocking the sperm from reaching your womb or Fallopian tubes

- blocking an embryo's journey down the Fallopian tubes

- preventing blood from flowing to your womb, meaning the endometrial lining doesn't thicken properly.

However, you can have fibroids and it not affect your fertility at all, so your fertility doctor may tell you that you have one or some but no treatment is necessary.

There are three types:

1. Subserous – grow on the outside wall of your womb

2. Intramural – grow in the muscle wall of your womb

3. Submucous – grow from the inner wall of your womb.

You may or may not have symptoms. Symptoms vary from heavy periods, swelling in your abdomen and pain and pressure in your pelvis. Diagnosis is by an ultrasound scan, hysteroscopy, laparoscopy or MRI scan.

Treatment depends on where the fibroids are, how big they are and how many there are. If you don't have any symptoms or your symptoms are mild, you may not need any treatment. Over the counter painkillers may help to ease pain. To reduce heavy bleeding, you may be prescribed medication or hormones, and to shrink them you may also be prescribed hormones. If you need surgery, an operation called a myomectomy will remove the fibroids but your womb will be left in place – this is the surgical choice if you want to get pregnant in the future. If your fibroids are on the inside wall of your womb, you may be advised to have a procedure called an endometrial ablation – removal of the lining of your womb which helps to reduce heavy bleeding. A procedure that shrinks the fibroid by blocking its blood supply is called uterine artery embolisation or UAE.

First Morning Urine – FMU

This is the very first pee you do in the morning on getting up when you are testing for ovulation or pregnancy. When you are using an ovulation predictor test (OPT) that relies on your pee to find out when you ovulate, you should use the first pee you do in the morning as it is the most valuable because it has more concentration of hormones. When you do the test, pee a little into the toilet first, then collect some pee into the container you use for the test.

When you are doing a home pregnancy test or HPT, providing you haven't done a pee in the night, the first morning urine will have a higher concentration of the pregnancy hormone hCG (human chorionic gonadotropin), meaning you get an accurate result sooner than if you used your pee from another time in the day or evening.

First Response Early Result Test – FRER
and Fertility Response Early Detection – FRED

This is the brand name of a make of home pregnancy test (HPT) and it claims to be able to detect the pregnancy hormone hCG (human chorionic gonadotropin) at least six days before your period is due. As with all HPTs, beware that you can get false positives especially if you test early. The only reliable pregnancy test is having a blood test done that gives a result as to how much hCG there is in your blood. I do not endorse this product nor do I have any association with the company. I have included it because the abbreviation is often seen on forums etc.

Folate

This should be part of the baseline blood test/blood work you have done in order to check your levels. In the UK, the Department of Health recommends that if you are trying to conceive, you should take a folic acid supplement of 400 mcg daily as well as eat a folate rich diet. This is likely the same advice in the country you live in. Low levels are a cause of anaemia. If you do not have adequate levels and you get pregnant, your baby is at risk of neural tube defects, such as spina bifida and anencephaly.

If you have the MTHFR gene mutation, you shouldn't take folic acid supplements – see 'Methylenetetrahydrofolate Reductase' for more information.

In men, correct folate levels are important for normal sperm health production and amount.

Follicle

This is a small fluid-filled sac which forms part of your ovary, and inside the follicle attached to the inner wall is an immature egg that may eventually mature. There are also cells in the follicle that produce the hormone oestrogen/estrogen which is needed for the egg to mature.

During your menstrual cycle several follicles begin to develop, as do the immature eggs, until ovulation occurs, when normally only one mature follicle with a mature egg erupts and releases the egg into your Fallopian tube. This is ovulation.

This empty follicle then turns into a 'corpus luteum' which also produces oestrogen/estrogen, and the hormone progesterone which thickens your womb lining ready for implantation, if the egg is fertilised. If the egg isn't fertilised, the corpus luteum turns into a 'corpus albicans', which is a fibrous scar on the ovary.

During the beginning of fertility treatment, your follicles are on your mind constantly because the hormone medication you take is designed to stimulate your ovaries and make them work overtime, in order to make lots of mature follicles and eggs for egg collection/retrieval. During this time, you will have regular ultrasounds to see how many follicles are growing on each ovary and what their size is, and the dosage of the medication will be changed as necessary. This is always a nerve-wracking time because everyone wants tons of good size follicles, but remember, it's not just about quantity – quality is also as important.

The below is not to scale and is an artistic impression of how the follicles change up to and including ovulation.

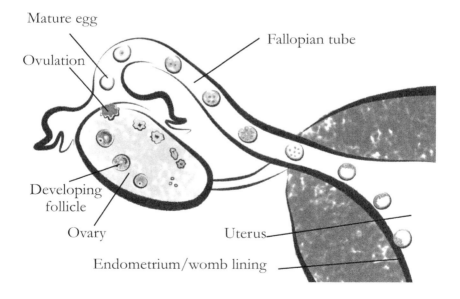

Follicle-Stimulating Hormone – FSH

This hormone is released by the pituitary gland in your brain, and is essential for normal functioning ovaries – mainly stimulating the growth of follicles in your ovaries, and ovulation; and in men, for normal sperm production.

Your levels of FSH vary throughout your menstrual cycle, with levels being at the highest immediately before ovulation. You may be wondering what the 'normal level' of FSH in your blood is – I'm afraid like most things where fertility is concerned, you will find varying answers as to what is 'normal'; this is due to laboratories having their own 'normal' values. But having a general idea of what is 'normal' will enable you to have a better discussion with your fertility specialist. A guideline is that during the follicular phase (see term below) and the luteal phase, the level should be in the range of 5-20 IU/L (international units per litre), and immediately before ovulation, the FSH level should be 30-50 IU/L.

The FSH level is also used to get an idea of your ovarian reserve by a blood test carried out on Day 3 of your cycle and, again, levels may vary but roughly under 6 IU/L is excellent, 6-9 IU/L is good, 9-10 IU/L is fair and 10-13 IU/L is classed as diminished ovarian reserve – see 'Diminished Ovarian Reserve' for more information.

Follicular Phase – FP

This is the second phase in your menstrual cycle – the first being menstruation which is when you bleed. The follicular phase lasts from Cycle Day 1 to Cycle Day 13 if you have an average menstrual cycle of 28 days, or up to ovulation if your cycle is longer or shorter.

What happens in this phase is the following:

1. The hypothalamus, in the brain, prompts the pituitary gland, also in the brain, to release follicle-stimulating hormone, or FSH.

2. FSH stimulates the ovary to produce a number of follicles – in each follicle is an immature egg cell, and one follicle and one egg cell mature.

3. At the same time as the follicle is maturing, the hormone oestrogen/estrogen is produced from the ovaries which builds up and thickens your womb lining, or endometrium, in order to receive a fertilised egg.

4. At ovulation, the mature follicle ruptures and the mature egg is released into the Fallopian tube. The last five days of this phase plus the day of ovulation are your 'fertile window'.

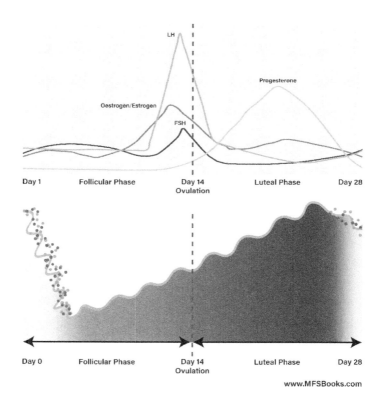

138

Fragmentation

If you are doing fertility treatment such as IVF, this is something you will hear at your clinic and it is another hurdle to jump over to get your baby. It's also called 'blebbing' and I have seen the term 'fragged-out' – I'm not sure which term is worse.

Fragmentation happens often (even in natural pregnancies though no one sees it), and is when small bits of cell material break off when the embryo is dividing. The fragments don't contain any genetic information and are just part of the jelly-like fluid that makes up all the cells in our bodies.

Usually an embryo that isn't dividing evenly and as expected has more fragmentation than one that is dividing evenly. Between fertilisation and when your embryo is transferred to your womb or is frozen, your embryos are graded and the embryo that is graded the best will be the one that is transferred as it is believed that it will give you the best chance of getting pregnant. See 'Embryo Grading' for more information.

It's important to know that once the embryo is transferred no one knows what happens and many, many times embryos with very little fragmentation unfortunately do not go on to make a baby. and the reason why was probably nothing to do with the lack of fragmentation. Similarly, many, many embryos that had quite a bit of fragmentation do go on to make a baby.

Free Thyroxine – FT4

See 'Thyroid Gland' for more information.

Freeze All

This simply means all embryos (rather than just the best ones) are frozen immediately following egg collection/retrieval and fertilisation. A frozen embryo/s will then be thawed at some point in the future and if the thawing process is successful, it/they will be transferred to your womb. For certain women, this freeze all approach may be more successful than transferring the best embryo at the end of the IVF or ICSI cycle.

Freezing Ovarian Tissue

Also called 'cryopreservation' of ovarian tissue, this is still an experimental method of preserving your fertility and is mostly carried out if you have cancer and will be undergoing treatment and would like to get pregnant in the future. It can be carried out quite quickly compared to egg freezing because tissue is being frozen rather than mature eggs.

What happens is that a part of an ovary or the whole ovary is removed during surgery, called a laparoscopy. Then the ovary's outer layer, the ovarian cortex which contains hundreds to thousands of immature eggs, is cut into small strips and frozen. When you are ready to have children, these ovarian strips are thawed and re-implanted and the immature eggs should start to develop normally.

You may be able to get pregnant naturally afterwards or you may need IVF. There have been babies born following ovarian freezing.

Frozen Embryo – Frostie

This is an embryo that developed during an IVF or ICSI cycle that is of good quality and a good grade and is expected to freeze well, then thaw so that it can be transferred to your womb in the future and hopefully become your baby. Providing it does freeze and thaw as expected, it has just as much chance of becoming a baby as an embryo that hasn't been frozen. See 'Embryo Cryopreservation/ Freezing' for more information.

Frozen Embryo Transfer – FET

This is when a frozen embryo is thawed and, if it thaws successfully, you will go to the clinic and have the embryo transferred in exactly the same way as a fresh embryo is transferred. See 'Embryo Transfer' for more information.

At the time of freezing the embryos, no one can predict which embryos will survive the freezing and the thawing process and which won't, and sadly, sometimes none survive, which can be extremely distressing as you have geared yourself up for your embryo/s to be transferred.

In the UK, so this is probably the same in other countries too, the success rates for IVF using frozen embryos have been increasing year on year and are now very similar to IVF using fresh embryos. In 2016, in women over 37 years old, birth rates for frozen embryo transfers (where the embryo was made from the woman's own eggs), were more successful than fresh embryo transfers with the woman's own embryos. The reason for this may be because the frozen embryos were made from her eggs when she was younger.

For some reasons, such as OHSS, you will be advised to not have any embryos transferred there and then because it is too dangerous, so all good quality embryos will be frozen. Another reason could be if you have raised progesterone levels after egg collection/ retrieval because this will affect the quality of your endometrium, so it would be in your interest to have either all your embryos frozen, known as 'freeze-all', or only the better-quality embryos frozen. Then the clinic can ensure your endometrium is the best it can be for a transfer at a later date.

Some fertility experts believe that for some women it may be more successful to have frozen embryos transferred at a later time because it gives her body the chance to recover from all the drugs she has taken and also allows her womb to calm down, so they would transfer a thawed embryo during her natural menstrual cycle.

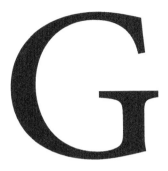

GAMETE INTRAFALLOPIAN TRANSFER

to

GYNAECOLOGIST

1 in 100 men have no sperm in their semen.

Gamete Intrafallopian Transfer – GIFT

This ART procedure was an early form of IVF. The ovaries were stimulated and the eggs collected/retrieved and mixed with the sperm. Then almost straight away, using laparoscopy, the egg and sperm mix was transferred using a soft plastic catheter, into one of the Fallopian tubes, where hopefully one egg would be fertilised. This isn't carried out any more as IVF is more successful.

Genetic Testing – GT

Also known as DNA testing, this is carried out for a number of reasons. One reason you may decide to have this test is if you are struggling to get pregnant, in order to determine if you or your partner (if you are using his sperm), are a carrier of a genetic condition that could be causing you to miscarry, and/or that could be passed onto any children you have. The test is carried out on a blood or a tissue sample.

Gestational Sac

This is what the embryo starts their life in and can be seen on ultrasound at approximately three to five weeks old. It is the first indication that there is a baby growing and if you have a scan at around six weeks (which a lot of us want to do after fertility treatment), you should see inside the yolk sac and see your baby with a heartbeat. So exciting!

Gestational Surrogacy/Carrier

This is a woman who carries a baby for another couple/woman but she is not the biological mother of the child and is not genetically related to the child. An egg from the biological mother and sperm from the father are combined using IVF or a variation of it, and then the fertilised embryo is transferred to the womb of the gestational surrogate/carrier. Alternatively, donor egg and/or donor sperm may be used.

The IVF cycle can either be when a fresh embryo is transferred to the surrogate, in which case the intended mother and the surrogate have to have their menstrual cycles synchronised, or the embryos are frozen after fertilisation and then thawed at a later date and transferred into the surrogate.

A gestational surrogate/carrier would be an option:

- if you don't have a womb
- if you have been through many ART treatments and still do not have your baby
- if you are at serious health risk yourself if you get pregnant, such as if you have a heart condition
- if the couple are gay men.

Some people who need to use a surrogate may ask a family member or a friend, and this can work very well as you all obviously know each other. If, however, you need to look further, there are agencies in many countries which allow surrogacy, and each country will have its own laws and regulations. You will need a lawyer who is familiar with the surrogacy laws and the costs of using a surrogate vary greatly from country to country. If you do travel abroad, getting a passport and the baby back into the UK, for example, can be a difficult and time-consuming process. In most countries you will need to apply for a parental order when you return with your baby/babies to the country that you live in. This is because the surrogate is recognised as the legal parent.

It goes without saying that neither the intended parent/s or surrogate go into surrogacy without giving it a lot of thought first as there is so much to consider. Everyone involved should receive counselling before, during and after the birth, and be open and honest about their expectations and what they don't want to happen. However, if done correctly and sensibly, it can give everyone involved a lot of pleasure and a future they only dreamed of.

See 'Surrogacy' for more information.

Ghost Lines

This is where, when doing a home pregnancy test (HPT) there are two lines but the second line is very faint and usually shows or becomes clearer after the allotted time the test tells you to check for the result. Therefore, if the test says 'Within 10 minutes a second line will display if you are pregnant' and you only see one very dark line (this line indicates the test is working), but you still check an hour later, the second line will be an evaporation or 'ghost line' of the darker first line.

This can be really frustrating and you don't know if you are pregnant or not. The best advice is to do another test a couple of days later – if you can wait that long – or have a blood test done as this is more accurate.

Gonadotropin-releasing Hormone – GnRH

This is produced in the hypothalamus in your brain. The hormone is carried in the blood to your pituitary gland, also in your brain where it stimulates the production of follicle-stimulating hormone (FSH) and luteinising hormone (LH) – two hormones important to fertility as they are responsible for maturing and releasing an egg, and in men, controlling the production of sperm.

Gynaecologist – Gynae

A doctor who has completed additional training in reproductive diseases in women.

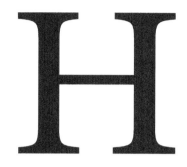

HAEMOSPERMIA

to

HYSTEROSALPINGOGRAM

The first successful IVF treatment was carried out because the mum had blocked Fallopian tubes.

Haemospermia or Haematospermia

This is blood in a man's semen or ejaculate. Understandably it causes him concern because it isn't normal, but it is rare and is more often caused by a urinary tract infection (UTI) or a sexually transmitted disease (STD), such as cytomegalovirus or chlamydia, which are easily treated.

If the infection is not treated it can cause damage to the reproductive system which could impact the man's fertility. If the cause is due to an STD it could be passed onto you which could then affect your fertility. In very rare cases the cause is due to cancer of the prostate.

Hashimoto's Thyroiditis – Hashi's

This was first explained in 1912 by a Japanese doctor and it is a cause of hypothyroidism (underactive thyroid gland located in your neck), specifically caused by autoimmunity – your body's autoimmune system attacks your thyroid gland causing inflammation. What causes Hashimoto's isn't known, but:

- it does tend to occur in families
- it is more common in women than in men
- it can be associated with type 1 diabetes and coeliac disease
- it can be triggered by stress and pregnancy.

As a result of being attacked, your thyroid gland does not produce enough thyroid hormones – thyroxine or T4 and triiodothyronine or T3. The symptoms of Hashimoto's are the same for hypothyroidism and are associated with a slowing metabolism (less energy).

It is diagnosed by:

- your symptoms and family medical history
- if you have a swelling in your neck because of an enlarged thyroid gland (a goitre)
- a blood test to check your thyroid-stimulating hormone (TSH) levels which will affect your T3 and T4 levels
- a blood test for antibodies, specifically anti-thyroperoxidase antibodies.

There is no cure for Hashimoto's thyroiditis and because it causes inflammation of the thyroid gland, hypothyroidism is inevitable. You will therefore be prescribed thyroid hormone medication which is a synthetic form of T4 (thyroxine) to alleviate the symptoms of hypothyroidism. You should have regular blood tests to check your TSH levels especially if you are trying to get pregnant, as your medication may need to be adjusted. If you have Hashimoto's thyroiditis you may have difficulty getting pregnant due to the symptoms of hypothyroidism. See 'Hypothyroidism' for more information.

History – Hx

In order to properly diagnose or to get a better idea of what may be happening that is preventing you from getting pregnant, you will be asked questions about your medical history, in the past and present. Often these questions are intrusive and private but unfortunately the fertility specialist does have to ask them to be able to decide what happens next, and which tests and/or investigations will help with a diagnosis. Where your fertility is concerned, if you are one half of a couple, your partner will have to provide their medical history too.

Home Pregnancy Test – HPT

This is the test we all can't wait to do following fertility treatment whilst at the same time dreading doing it. As its name suggests, it's a test you do at home to check if you are pregnant or not. The test works by detecting a hormone called human chorionic gonadotropin (hCG for short) in your pee, so basically you pee on a test stick, or into a container then put the test stick in the container. It is really important you follow the instructions carefully because if you don't, your result may not be accurate. Some brands of HPT are able to detect hCG in your urine sooner than others.

Most women will test to see if they are pregnant before the clinic advises, known as OTD (on test day); it is almost impossible not to. However, there is a reason the clinic advises this and it is because you could test too early and the HPT shows a negative result, so you think your fertility treatment hasn't worked when it actually has. You can save yourself a lot of heartache and anxiety by waiting a couple more days (I know it's hard) before you test.

Sheila says: I'll let you into a secret; on our third ICSI cycle (which was our successful one) I was too scared to do a HPT because I didn't want to see a negative result – you know the one, it says 'Not Pregnant'; talk about rub it in. So, I didn't test and went to our local hospital to have a blood test instead. Our clinic rang up later that day to find out our result because we hadn't rung the day before. I had got the dates wrong and had got the blood test done a day later than the clinic advised! I must be the only woman in the world to do a test later than advised!

Hormones

There are a number of hormones that are relevant to fertility and if a hormone level is not within a normal range, this is very likely to affect your ability to become pregnant and/or stay pregnant. All the following hormones are explained in greater detail elsewhere in this book, but in a nutshell:

- gonadotropin-releasing hormone (GnRH) causes the release of follicle-stimulating hormone (FSH) and luteinising hormone (LH) in the pituitary gland. FSH stimulates the growth of follicles in your ovaries, and in men stimulates the production of sperm. LH brings about ovulation, and in men it activates the production of testosterone

- prolactin is produced in the pituitary gland and a very high level can prevent ovulation

- oestradiol/oestrogen is produced in the ovaries and in other parts of your body, and it causes your endometrium (womb lining) to grow during your menstrual cycle so that it is ready for a fertilised egg to implant

- progesterone, along with oestrogen/estrogen, prepares your endometrium to receive a fertilised egg

- thyroid-stimulating hormone (TSH) is produced in the pituitary gland and stimulates the thyroid gland to produce thyroxine or T3

- adrenaline, cortisol, testosterone and DHEA are all produced by the adrenal glands which sit on top of your kidneys.

See 'The miracle of Mother Nature' at the beginning of this book to read exactly what needs to happen and when to create a baby.

The two following illustrations are not to scale and are an artistic impression of the glands that are involved with your, and male, fertility hormones.

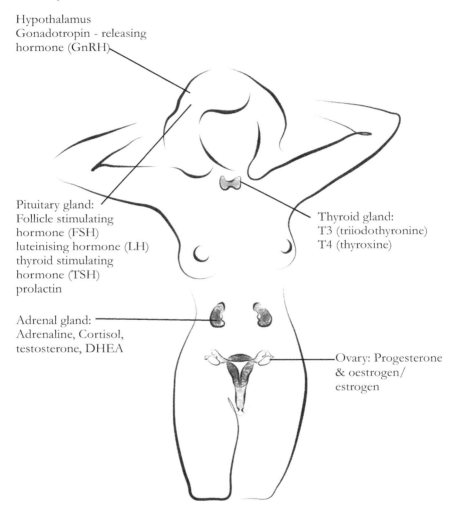

Hypothalamus
Gonadotropin - releasing
hormone (GnRH)

Pituitary gland:
Follicle stimulating
hormone (FSH)
luteinising hormone (LH)
thyroid stimulating
hormone (TSH)
prolactin

Thyroid gland:
T3 (triiodothyronine)
T4 (thyroxine)

Adrenal gland:
Adrenaline, Cortisol,
testosterone, DHEA

Ovary: Progesterone
& oestrogen/
estrogen

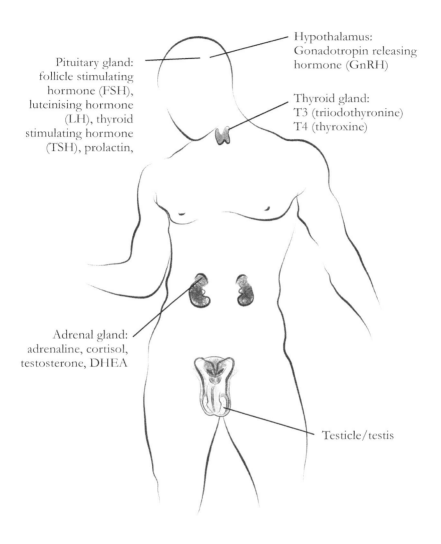

Pituitary gland: follicle stimulating hormone (FSH), luteinising hormone (LH), thyroid stimulating hormone (TSH), prolactin,

Hypothalamus: Gonadotropin releasing hormone (GnRH)

Thyroid gland: T3 (triiodothyronine) T4 (thyroxine)

Adrenal gland: adrenaline, cortisol, testosterone, DHEA

Testicle/testis

Hughes Syndrome

See 'Anti-phospholipid Syndrome' for more information.

Human Chorionic Gonadotropin – hCG

When you are doing fertility treatment such as IVF or ICSI, after your ovaries have been stimulated to produce multiple follicles, the last injection you do before your egg collection/retrieval (EC/ER) contains this hormone, and it matures the eggs that have been developing in the follicles.

The timing of this injection is crucial because your EC/ER must be done when a certain number of hours have passed. The injection is usually done late at night, and around 36 hours later, in the morning, you have your EC/ER. The main side effect of this medication is that it can cause some women to develop a condition called OHSS, which can be life threatening if left untreated. See 'Ovarian Hyperstimulation Syndrome' for more information.

hCG is also referred to as the 'pregnancy hormone' because it is made during pregnancy by cells in the placenta once the embryo has implanted. Levels of hCG can first be measured in a blood test approximately 11 days after conception or, if doing a home pregnancy test (HPT), which is when you pee on a stick, 12-14 days after conception. An hCG level of less than 5mIU/ml (milli-international units per millilitre) is considered a negative pregnancy result and anything above 25mIU/ml is considered a positive pregnancy result. The hCG level doubles every 48-72 hours until 8-11 weeks of pregnancy when it declines and levels off for the remainder of the pregnancy.

Sheila says: On forums, if you get a positive pregnancy test you'll see 'BFP' which stands for 'Big Fat Positive'. If, unfortunately, your test is negative, it's written as 'BFN', which stands for 'Big Fat Negative'.

Human Fertilisation & Embryology Authority – HFEA

This is the UK Government's independent regulator overseeing fertility treatment and research. Their impartial information for fertility patients is free and includes information about:

- fertility clinics in the UK
- NHS funding
- egg donation
- sperm donation
- fertility treatments
- preserving your fertility
- surrogacy
- genetic diseases.

Humira

This is a treatment you may be prescribed by your fertility clinic if it is believed that you have an autoimmune condition (where your body fights healthy cells), that is stopping you from getting pregnant. Humira was manufactured to treat certain severe forms of arthritis (which is an autoimmune disease), and some bowel disorders. There have been no evidence-based studies done on whether it is an effective fertility treatment so the use of it to treat infertility is still controversial and you need to do your own research.

Hydrosalpinx

This is when a Fallopian tube is blocked at the ovary end and contains fluid. Sometimes both tubes can be affected and this is called 'hydrosalpinges'. The tube appears swollen, similar to a sausage, due to the fluid. More often than not you don't know you have hydrosalpinx as there are rarely symptoms, though some women experience pelvic pain. It's likely you would only find out you have hydrosalpinx during investigations if you are trying to get pregnant.

The cause is usually due to a long-term infection of the Fallopian tube, such as:

- a sexually transmitted disease (STD)
- ruptured appendix
- pelvic inflammatory disease (PID) affecting the uterus, ovaries or vagina.

It can also be caused by adhesions or by endometriosis.

Diagnosis is by a hysterosalpingogram (HSG) but to determine if the blockage is definitely due to a hydrosalpinx, you may need a sonohysterosalpingography. Alternatively, a laparoscopy may be performed to diagnose.

You may be advised to have the tube surgically drained or have a salpingectomy, which is when the tube is surgically removed. Antibiotics may also be prescribed for the infection.

Hyperprolactinaemia

This is when there is too much of the hormone prolactin in your blood. Prolactin is produced by the brain's pituitary gland and it regulates your menstrual periods and helps your breasts to grow and produce breast milk when you're pregnant. A high level reduces oestrogen/estrogen, which affects ovulation, which in turn causes irregular or absent periods and can cause infertility.

Men also produce prolactin and high levels can cause low levels of testosterone, low sperm count and impotence.

Often the cause is unknown but it can be caused by:

- a non-cancerous tumour in the pituitary gland

- overactive cells in the pituitary gland

- underactive thyroid – see 'Hypothyroidism' for more information

- certain medications, such as some medications for depression and high blood pressure.

It is diagnosed by a blood test and an MRI scan of your brain.

Treatment is by medication, or if a large tumour is the cause, surgery will be carried out.

Once your prolactin level has returned to normal it is very likely that you will start to ovulate again and the man's sperm count will improve.

Hyperthyroidism

This is when your thyroid gland, located in your neck, is overactive and produces too much of the thyroid hormones thyroxine (T4) and triiodothyronine (T3), and can be due to the following:

- Graves' disease, also known as Basedow's disease

- enlarged thyroid gland (goitre)

- inflammation of the thyroid gland

- taking too much medication for hypothyroidism.

The symptoms of hyperthyroidism are due to an increase in the body's metabolism (energy) and include:

- palpitations/rapid pulse
- tiredness and weak muscles
- irritability and nervousness (hyperactivity)
- weight loss but increase in appetite
- anxiety
- sensitivity to high temperatures and sweating
- shakiness
- warm moist hands
- hair loss
- thyroid eye disease – bulging eyes that are gritty and sore.

Hyperthyroidism affects your fertility in the following ways:

- irregular menstrual cycles
- lack of periods (amenorrhea)
- loss of libido.

Hyperthyroidism in men is rarer than in women and it affects their fertility because of high levels of hormones, especially testosterone, which can affect sperm production and quality.

Treatment is by anti-thyroid medication, surgery, radioactive iodine and making lifestyle and diet changes. Once your thyroid gland is functioning normally, there is no reason why you shouldn't get pregnant naturally providing there are no other conditions that could be causing your infertility.

Hypnotherapy

This is a complimentary therapy and some people believe it helps you to get pregnant if you have been trying and nothing has happened; but this is inconclusive. Hypnotherapy helps you go into an altered state of consciousness, like being in a trance. Your mind is active though your body is deeply relaxed. You will know where you are and what is happening to you and you will remember it afterwards.

It can help replace negative beliefs and thoughts with positive ones. Some research indicates that the deep relaxation part can help you to feel less stressed. It is thought that it may help to reduce levels of the hormone prolactin, which hinders ovulation.

Hypogonadism

This is when the sex glands, which are the ovaries or testes/testicles, produce little or no sex hormone. Sex hormones help to control secondary sexual characteristics and also play a role in your menstrual cycle and, in men, in sperm production.

The cause may be due to:

- a problem with the ovaries or testicles
- the pituitary gland or hypothalamus not functioning correctly
- autoimmune disorder
- severe infection
- radiation treatment.

The symptoms you may experience include:

- lack of menstruation
- loss of body hair
- a lack of or reduced libido.

In men, symptoms include:

- loss of body hair
- muscle loss
- abnormal breast growth
- low or absent sex drive and
- infertility due to a reduced sperm count.

It is diagnosed by testing the levels of follicle-stimulating hormone (FSH) and luteinising hormone (LH) in both of you, and also the levels of oestrogen/estrogen for you and testosterone for him. Your male partner will also have to provide a semen sample in order to check the sperm count.

Other blood tests may include checking if either of you are anaemic (as iron levels can affect production of the sex hormones), prolactin hormone levels and thyroid levels.

Treatment for both of you includes hormone therapy or if the problem is caused by a tumour on the pituitary gland, this will be treated.

Hypothalamus

This is a gland in your brain and is the link between your nervous system and endocrine system – which is important for your reproduction. The hormone that is secreted by the hypothalamus and which is concerned with fertility is gonadotropin releasing hormone or GnRH, which stimulates the secretion of follicle-stimulating hormone (FSH) and luteinising hormone (LH).

In you, FSH stimulates the growth of follicles in your ovaries and in men it stimulates the production of sperm. LH in you brings about ovulation and in men it activates the production of testosterone.

Hypothalamic Amenorrhea

This is a condition in which menstruation ceases for several months due to the hypothalamus (a gland in your brain), not producing the hormone GnRH (Gonadotropin-releasing Hormone), which results in the amount of FSH (follicle stimulating hormone) and LH (luteinising hormone) dropping which causes menstruation and ovulation to stop, resulting in infertility. It can be caused by:

- high levels of stress

- excessive exercising

- weight loss

- coming off birth control pills

- eating disorders.

By making lifestyle changes your menstruation and ovulation should return providing you have no other medical issues.

Hypothyroidism

This is when your thyroid gland, located in your neck, is underactive and doesn't produce enough of the hormones thyroxine (T4) and triiodothyronine (T3). It can be caused by:

- autoimmune thyroid disease, where the body's immune

system attacks the thyroid gland; the commonest is Hashimoto's thyroiditis – see this term for more information

- radioactive thyroid treatment to correct hyperthyroidism

- too much anti-thyroid medication being taken for hyperthyroidism

- side effect of some medications taken for other disorders

- pituitary gland not functioning normally

- eating too much of some health foods that contain iodine.

Symptoms of hypothyroidism often begin gradually and you don't notice them until it is quite advanced. They include:

- slow heart rate

- raised cholesterol

- fatigue

- depression

- irritability

- dry/rough skin

- constipation

- feeling cold even when the environment is warm

- poor appetite or weight gain and

- low libido.

Often you don't know you have hypothyroidism until you have your thyroid-stimulating hormone (TSH) and T3 and T4 levels tested.

Hypothyroidism affects your fertility negatively in the following ways:

- reduces follicle-stimulating hormone (FSH) and luteinising hormone (LH) levels, which are required for maturing the egg follicles

- causes irregular menstrual cycles

- makes your periods heavy and longer

- causes you to have low basal body temperature (BBT)

- increases your chance of miscarriages.

If a man has hypothyroidism this can also affect his fertility in the following ways:

- high levels of thyroid-stimulating hormone or TSH in his bloodstream can cause his prolactin hormone levels to be high

- low testosterone levels due to high prolactin levels can result in a fall in the amount of sperm being produced, as well as causing erectile dysfunction and a low sex drive.

Medical treatment for both of you is to take a thyroxine drug. Focusing on foods that are good for the thyroid and certain herbs are also believed to help but you must discuss this with your doctor.

Hystero-Salpingo Contrast Sonography – HyCoSy

Also referred to as a saline contrast ultrasound, this is similar to a hysterosalpingogram as to why and how it is done. It is performed to check for major uterine abnormalities such as:

- polycystic ovaries (PCO)

- fibroids

- polyps

- uterine septa and

- other problems in the pelvis, as well as checking that your Fallopian tubes are open.

The main difference between this and the hysterosalpingogram explained below, are the cost to have it done, and that the fluid used in the HyCoSy is saline but iodine in the hysterosalpingogram.

Hysterosalpingogram

This procedure is carried out to look at your womb and to find out if your Fallopian tubes are open or blocked and, if blocked, where the blockage is. It will be done between Days 1 and 14 of your menstrual cycle. It uses an X-ray and takes less than five minutes and you won't need any anaesthetic. It is similar to a smear/PAP smear.

A thin tube is inserted through your cervix using a speculum and then passed into your womb. Liquid iodine is passed through the tube. The iodine shows up your womb and Fallopian tubes on the X-ray. Images are taken showing how the fluid is moving around your womb and through your Fallopian tubes. You may experience cramping and discomfort during the procedure and afterwards, along with dizziness.

If the report shows that there is a blockage in your Fallopian tube(s), you may need a procedure called a laparoscopy, which is more in depth.

The below is not to scale and is an artistic impression of a hysterosalpingogram.

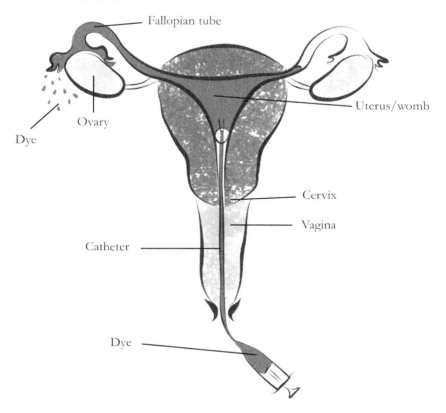

Hysteroscopy – HSC

This is a procedure used to look inside your womb using a narrow telescope with a light and camera called a hysteroscope. It is carried out in the same way as a smear/PAP smear – a speculum is passed into your vagina and cervix and the hysteroscope is passed through it into your womb.

A small amount of fluid is gently passed into your womb so the doctor or nurse can see inside more clearly. The images from the camera are viewed on a monitor. It takes about 10-15 minutes and is usually done without the need for any anaesthetic. Afterwards, you may experience cramping like period pains, spotting or bleeding for a couple of days and sex should be avoided until the bleeding has stopped, or for a week to reduce the risk of infection.

It is carried out:

- to diagnose conditions such as fibroids and polyps
- to investigate symptoms or problems such as heavy periods or pelvic pain
- to treat conditions and problems such as removing fibroids, polyps or uterine adhesions.

The below is not to scale and is an artistic impression of your reproductive system.

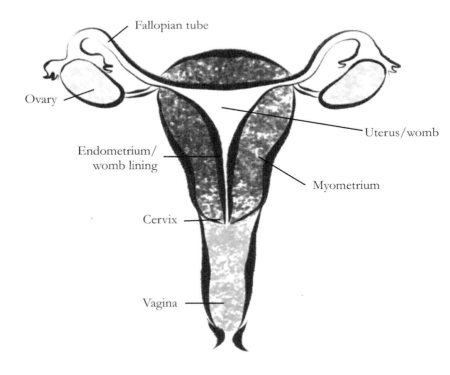

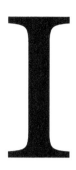

IMMATURE OOCYTE/EGG RETRIEVAL to IVF NATURAL CYCLE

The first IVF baby in the world was born in the UK on 25 July 1978; her name is Louise Brown. Her younger sister Natalie Brown was the fourth baby. Natalie was the first IVF baby to have a baby, in 1999, and she conceived naturally.

Immature Oocyte/Egg Retrieval – IOR

The 'immature' refers to underdeveloped eggs being retrieved or collected during ART such as IVF rather than your eggs being collected too early in the IVF cycle. Up until the actual retrieval, the doctor won't be aware that some or all of your eggs are immature because your follicles could be growing as expected.

The cause of your eggs not maturing maybe due to the drug that was used for your stimulation was unsuitable for you, especially if you are older, or you have reduced ovarian reserve or PCOS.

The below is not to scale and is an artistic impression of egg collection/retrieval procedure.

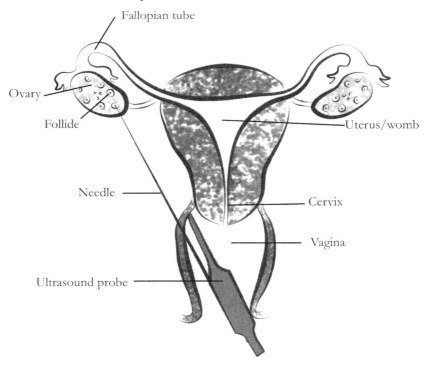

Immune Therapy

This is more often thought of when you have had recurrent failed IVF cycles but, if you have had a number of miscarriages at eight to ten weeks pregnant naturally, you may want to look into being tested for immune issues, and depending on the results, you may require treatment.

This is a controversial area where fertility is concerned with some fertility experts believing immune treatment benefits some women, and other experts claiming there is not enough evidence to prove these treatments work. Please do your research and ask questions and seek a second opinion if this is something you want to know more about. See 'Intralipid' and/or 'Intravenous Immunoglobulin G infusion – IVIg' for more information.

Implantation

When an egg is fertilised by a sperm and arrives in your womb, either naturally or with a bit of outside help, for you to get pregnant it needs to implant into a womb lining that is willing and able to develop it into a baby – this is known as the 'implantation window'. In a natural pregnancy, implantation occurs around Day 20-24 of your menstrual cycle, which is 6-12 days post ovulation or 'dpo' – as is commonly written on forums. If you have had IVF for example, with a Day 5 blastocyst transfer, implantation should occur one to two days after your transfer; with a Day 2 or 3 embryo transfer, it will be between 6-10 days after your egg collection/retrieval.

If you are doing a frozen embryo transfer or FET, your transfer will be during a fresh cycle. This may be during your natural cycle, in which case the clinic will synchronise your transfer according to how many days your embryo is with the correct days in your cycle, ensuring your endometrium is at the correct stage to receive your embryo. Or you will still take medication to thicken your womb lining, have scans to measure the thickness and then start taking progesterone medication to make the lining ready for implantation, and the transfer is done approximately five days later.

For implantation to be successful following IVF and other similar treatments, the embryo or blastocyst that is transferred needs to be of a good quality and your uterine lining needs to be at least 7-8mm on transfer day. The hormone progesterone, produced by your ovaries, is important for making your lining very receptive which is why you are prescribed it following egg collection/retrieval.

Having a well-balanced diet and drinking lots of fluid for at least three months prior to starting your treatment is highly recommended rather than cramming yourself full of 'superfoods' just before your treatment starts. Think of your uterine lining as the soil in a field and your embryo as the seed – seeds develop much better in great quality, squishy soil than dry, poor quality soil.

After fertility treatment, your focus changes again from how many eggs have fertilised to 'has my embryo implanted?' Oh, for a see-through tummy! For more information and advice – see 'Two-Week Wait' further on in this book.

Implantation Bleed – IB

This can be mistaken for the beginning of your menstrual period. In some of us, when the fertilised egg implants into the endometrium it causes a slight bleed. The blood loss is usually very minimal and is usually a pinky/brown colour. It may last for a couple of hours or one to two days and is often referred to as 'spotting'. It will stop on its own and is not harmful to the baby. It is an early sign of pregnancy and after having fertility treatment, such as IVF, during the two-week wait, a lot of us obsess about this because it is a 'sign'. If we don't get this 'sign' we think we're not pregnant when in fact we missed it because it was so slight.

Implantation Failure

This is when your embryo (or embryos) fails to implant into your womb after fertility treatment such as IVF, and you get a negative pregnancy test. This is so very upsetting and frustrating after all you have been through. There are a number of reasons why this happens and we mostly blame ourselves – we did something wrong or we didn't do something that we should have. However, this is almost certainly not the case, as the cause is more often than not due to embryo quality or there may be an issue with your womb lining/endometrium.

Where the embryo is concerned:

- it may have looked like a good quality embryo in the laboratory but it stopped developing once it was transferred, and this is usually due to chromosomal abnormalities
- there may be genetic abnormalities of the egg or the sperm; in these embryos they don't produce a chemical that signals to the uterine lining to get prepared for implantation.

Your womb lining needs to be ready to receive an embryo and if it isn't, for any reason, implantation won't happen; it's very similar to the window of opportunity for fertilisation – if there are no sperm hanging around when you ovulate, fertilisation won't happen. Problems with your womb lining could be due to:

- infection of the endometrium – for example, if due to Tuberculosis (TB) this is quite common if you come from an area where TB is more prevalent

- if you have Asherman's syndrome where the walls of your womb stick together

- if your lining isn't thick enough – it should be more than 7 mm thick – which is often due to a lack of the hormone progesterone being produced. This is known as a 'luteal phase deficit' or LPD – see this term for more information

- if you have fibroids or adhesions which may prevent an embryo from implanting.

If it is believed you have implantation failure due to your womb lining, an investigation into the receptivity of your lining may be suggested – see 'Endometrial Receptivity Array Test' or ERA for more information.

Incubator

This is the first home for your future child if you are doing fertility treatment such as IVF or ICSI. The incubator in the laboratory at the fertility clinic looks a little like a domestic fridge, but the conditions inside mimic the inside of your womb in terms of the temperature, humidity and the amount of oxygen and carbon dioxide. On the door is your information so the embryologist knows whose eggs or embryos are inside without having to open the door, as each time the door is opened, it disturbs the eggs and embryos. Often the incubators are stacked on top of each other so that they can fit more in.

Like all things to do with fertility, technology is advancing all the time and some incubators may have cameras fitted to them to regularly take images of the developing embryos. There are also some that are the size of a champagne cork so that the developing embryos can fit inside your vagina.

Infertility – IF

The WHO (World Health Organisation) definition of infertility is 'a disease of the reproductive system defined by the failure to achieve a clinical pregnancy after 12 months or more of regular unprotected sexual intercourse'.

In the world around one in seven couples – that's 50 million couples and individuals – have difficulty in conceiving – though this number could be higher as many people still don't seek help. About 84% of couples will conceive naturally within one year if they have regular (every two or three days), unprotected sex.

There are two types of infertility:

1. primary is where a woman who's never conceived has difficulty conceiving

2. secondary, where a woman has had one or more pregnancies previously but is now having difficulty conceiving.

Intended Parent(s) in Surrogacy – IPS

These are couples or individuals who have tried for many years to become parents to their own biological child either naturally or through fertility treatment. If the IPS have frozen embryos they will often look at surrogacy in order to still have their own biological child. For some same-sex couples or a single man, they will turn to surrogacy straight away in order to have a biological child.

International Council on Infertility Information Dissemination – inciid

Pronounced 'inside', this is a non-profit organisation started in the USA in 1995 by three women affected by infertility. It is now global and helps individuals and couples explore the different options for having a family. They provide up-to-date information and support regarding diagnosis, treatment and prevention of infertility and pregnancy loss, and guidance if you are considering adoption or a child-free lifestyle.

Intracytoplasmic Morphological Selected Sperm Injection – IMSI

This is the same as ICSI the next term, and therefore similar to IVF, but a high-power microscope is used which magnifies each sperm up to around 1500 times enabling the embryologist to select sperm with what appears to be a normal-looking nucleus.

Intracytoplasmic Sperm Injection – ICSI

This is the most common and successful fertility treatment where male factor is the cause, such as:

- low sperm count
- sperm with poor morphology (shape)
- sperm with poor motility (movement)
- if sperm has to be collected surgically from the testicles/testes

- there were problems with fertilisation in previous IVF cycles.

The success rate for ICSI is similar to IVF. The treatment is the same as for IVF from down-regulation, stimulation, up to and including egg collection/retrieval (EC/ER). Then, rather than putting sperm in a dish with an egg and letting them get on with the process of fertilisation, an embryologist uses a microscope to select a sperm that is swimming vigorously and in a straight line, from the sample provided by your husband/partner or a donor, and injects it into the egg using a very small needle. This may sound quite simple but it takes a lot of skill and the embryologist will have received further training after qualifying. The egg/sperm is then put into an incubator to allow fertilisation and development of the embryo – the same as with IVF. See 'In Vitro Fertilisation' for more information.

ICSI doesn't guarantee that fertilisation will happen, just that the sperm has entered the egg. There is usually, but not always, an additional cost on top of the costs for IVF.

The following illustration is not to scale and is an artistic impression of ICSI.

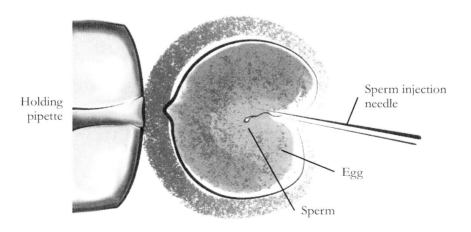

Holding pipette

Sperm injection needle

Egg

Sperm

Intralipid

This is an intravenous (meaning it's given into your blood) infusion of a fat emulsion given to people who have a fatty acid deficiency. The infusion contains soya bean oil, egg yolk, glycerine and water.

Some fertility experts believe it can help you to get pregnant if you have an abnormal immune response resulting in unexplained infertility, repeated IVF failures and recurrent miscarriage. Your immune system fights and destroys any foreign body that could be harmful to you, but if yours is 'abnormal', it also fights foreign cells that aren't harmful, such as an embryo. On the other hand, there are fertility experts who do not believe it helps and see this treatment as another way to build up your hopes.

Because it is quite a new 'treatment' for infertility it is difficult to find statistics from large trials and studies – as is always the case when something is new. You will read on forums that women have had babies following taking intralipids and you'll also read that some women have taken intralipids and haven't had a baby.

Intramuscular Injection – IM

Some medication used during fertility treatments such as IVF has to be given as an injection into muscle, so the usual sites for this are your thigh or your bum cheeks. The thought of injecting yourself usually freaks most people out and is one part of the cycle that really does cause worry and anxiety. It isn't a pleasant thing to do to yourself so many women get their partner or a friend to do it instead – even they aren't that keen on the idea of sticking a needle into you.

Your nurse at the clinic will explain and show you how to do it and often you do the first injection there with the nurse; typically, it goes fine at the clinic and it is only when you get home that you lose all confidence in yourself and think you can't do it. Your own clinic might have videos on their website that you can watch as often as you like at home, but if they don't, there are plenty of videos of how to do intramuscular injections on the internet.

Intrauterine Insemination – IUI

This procedure is where sperm are placed inside your womb to increase the chances of an egg being fertilised as more sperm will be near to your Fallopian tubes when you ovulate (release an egg) – so it should be carried out about 12 hours after ovulation. It is often recommended for:

- unexplained infertility
- male infertility
- hostile cervical mucus
- if pain during sex makes intercourse impossible
- if donor sperm is being used.

IUI may be carried out with or without fertility drugs. If you are taking fertility drugs such as Clomid, you will have ultrasound scans and blood tests prior to the IUI.

The IUI itself is carried out at the fertility clinic and although it is a simple procedure, you're still likely to feel nervous, excited and scared and this is perfectly normal. It shouldn't be painful and doesn't take long.

If you are using your partner's sperm, he will produce the semen sample first as the sperm have to be 'washed' to remove any impurities – see 'Sperm Washing' for more information. If you are using donor sperm it will be thawed first.

The below is not to scale and is purely an artistic impression of the procedure 'sperm washing.'

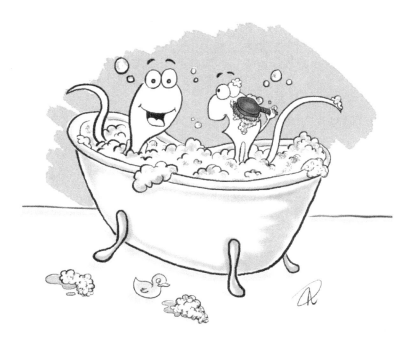

The procedure is similar to having a pap/smear done; a speculum is inserted into your vagina and a thin, plastic catheter is gently inserted through your vagina and into your cervix. The sperm is then passed through the catheter into your womb near to your Fallopian tubes. The catheter and speculum are then removed.

Most of us want to remain lying down for several hours to give the sperm a fighting chance of reaching our Fallopian tubes, but in most clinics, you will probably be able to lie down for 30 minutes or so. Try to fight doing a strange 'thigh-together-waddle' as you leave the room (tempting though it is) – the sperm were deposited into your womb and the only way to go… is up. You may be given progesterone medication to take until you do either a home pregnancy test or have a blood test to check your human chorionic gonadotropin (hCG) levels to see if you are pregnant.

IUI is significantly cheaper than IVF and is less risky if no fertility drugs are taken.

The below is not to scale and is an artistic impression of IUI.

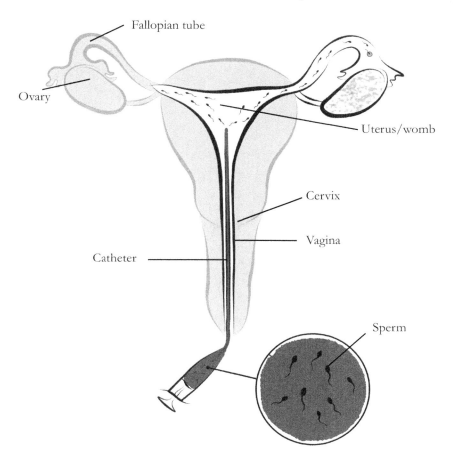

Intravaginal Insemination – IVI

Also known as artificial insemination, this is a technique often used for male infertility where your fertility is not compromised, or by lesbian couples or single women as it mimics what happens naturally during intercourse. It can be carried out at home or at a fertility clinic. It should be carried out about 12 hours after ovulation so home ovulation kits can be used or a blood test is taken for levels of the luteinising hormone (LH). If you have been on fertility drugs to stimulate your ovaries you will be monitored closely.

In the clinic the actual procedure takes about ten minutes and should be painless, though some discomfort may be experienced. A speculum is inserted into your vagina so that a fine plastic catheter (tube) can be passed into your cervix. A syringe with the sperm in is fitted to the catheter and the sperm are gently deposited through the catheter into your cervix. A sponge cap may be placed over the cervix to prevent the sperm from leaking out and you may be advised to lie down for 30 minutes.

At home, either a sterile syringe is used to get the sperm into your vagina or the sperm is placed inside a cervical cap and you put this as near to your cervix as possible.

Intravenous Immunoglobulin G Infusion – IVIg

This is a treatment that may be given to you if you have had recurrent miscarriages and/or implantation failures with ART, due to autoimmune factors such as natural killer cells (NK cells). See 'Natural Killer Cells' for more information. As with a lot of fertility treatments that are termed 'add-ons', there are the believers of this treatment and the non-believers – making it very hard for you to know what to do.

IVIg is a solution of human antibodies taken from donor blood and given via a saline infusion into your blood over two to four hours. The antibodies help to keep your immune system from recognising an embryo as a foreign body and attacking it.

There are side effects to the treatment and the severity depends on the amount you receive and for how long. Some side effects are:

- fever and chills
- nausea
- headache
- skin irritation at the site of the infusion.

It is an expensive treatment as you often have a treatment prior to getting pregnant or starting an ART cycle and then monthly thereafter and quite far into your pregnancy.

As with all fertility treatments, please do your research and speak to the specialists and get a second opinion if you're still unsure.

In Vitro Fertilisation – IVF

This is a general term used for fertilisation of an egg by a sperm that occurs outside of your body 'in vitro,' meaning 'in glass'. The first baby born successfully after IVF treatment was in 1978 in the UK. It is suitable for people with a wide range of fertility issues and for same-sex males who want their own biological family using a surrogate.

The main part of IVF is the same for all, though what drugs you take and the dosage is individual to you specifically. Also, how long a cycle is will depend on your precise protocol; you may do a long or a short/flat protocol, which means your treatment cycle can last for between three to six weeks.

There are also different types of IVF which are described in this book, namely 'IVF Mild' and 'IVF Natural'; the differences are to do with the amounts of drugs that are prescribed.

The first part of any IVF cycle is all do to with switching off your reproductive hormones, which is known as 'down regulation', so that your fertility doctor can take over control – see 'Down Regulation' for more information. It is more common that you follow the short or flat protocol these days which means the down regulation time is shorter and you take less medication.

If you do a long protocol cycle, you still down regulate but the period of time is longer and you take more medication as a nasal spray or injection.

The next phase is known as 'stimulation' and you will take fertility drugs to stimulate more follicles in your ovaries to develop and to produce mature eggs – see 'Stimulation' for more information. During this time, you are regularly monitored by ultrasound scan to check the number of follicles in your ovaries, their size and how thick your uterine lining (endometrium) is, and your blood is tested for your hormone levels. How many scans and blood tests you have varies from clinic to clinic and many clinics now open quite early in the morning which may be more convenient for you.

The last stage before egg collection/retrieval is the hCG or human chorionic gonadotropin injection, and this must be done around 36 hours before egg collection/retrieval as it matures the eggs.

Egg collection/retrieval is dreaded and anticipated in equal measures – it is what you have been so focused on and working towards since that first sniff or injection. It is done in the morning and it is performed usually under either sedation or local anaesthetic but still in an operating theatre. It can be uncomfortable and painful so you will probably be given pain relief beforehand. It takes about 30 minutes, and in some clinics your partner can be with you but check at your clinic beforehand so you both know what to expect. See 'Egg Collection/Retrieval' for more information.

The below is not to scale and is an artistic impression of an egg collection/retrieval procedure.

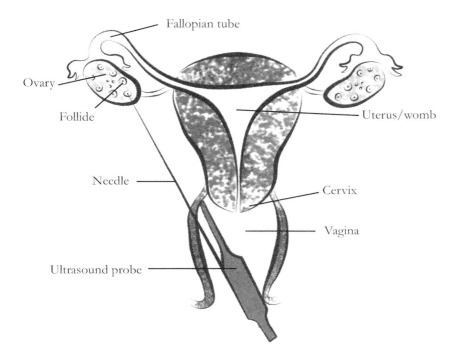

Fallopian tube

Ovary

Follide

Needle

Ultrasound probe

Uterus/womb

Cervix

Vagina

After egg collection/retrieval, whilst you are recovering, the embryologist examines each egg under the microscope. It is kept in its own plastic dish in a liquid called culture medium. The embryologist also looks at your partner's semen sample, if he has provided one before your egg collection. He/she checks the quality and quantity and then it is 'washed' to remove impurities and any dead or sluggish sperm – see 'Sperm Washing' for more information.

The sperm are then added to the eggs in their individual dishes and the dishes are put into the incubator where, hopefully, a sperm will fertilise the egg.

The below illustration is not to scale and is purely an artistic impression of IVF fertilisation.

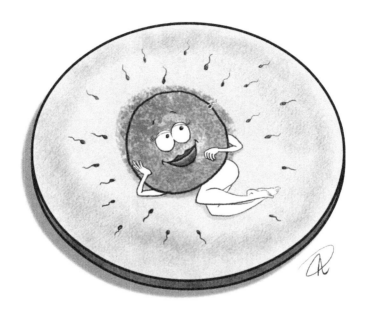

Now it's a horrible waiting game and your focus changes to how many of your eggs have fertilised and continue to develop. Usually the embryologist, but it could be the nurse, at your clinic phones you the next day to tell you how many eggs have fertilised – this is either good news or not very good news. If the latter this is very upsetting as we all assume all our eggs will fertilise. The embryologist regularly checks on the development of the fertilised eggs and again someone from the clinic calls you each day with an update until they decide when your embryo transfer will take place.

The next hurdle is the embryo or blastocyst transfer and this is really where you take the advice of your clinic rather than the advice on forums; sorry to say this. The transfer is either carried out on Day 2, Day 3 or Day 5 – when depends on how well your embryos are developing, and although most people want a Day 5 transfer, possibly because it is believed you are more likely to get pregnant, many babies are born following Day 2 (our daughter was), and Day 3 transfers. Your clinic knows you best, knows your treatment best so they are the best ones to advise you. Don't forget, they really want you to get pregnant and for you to hold your baby in your arms almost as much as you do. See 'Embryo Transfer' for more information.

The below is not to scale and is an artistic impression of embryo development. See 'Embryo Development' for more information.

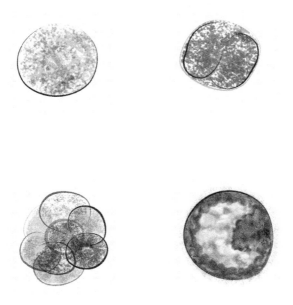

Then you have the dreaded, emotionally charged, rollercoaster two-week wait (TWW or 2WW) until you test to see if you are pregnant. Everyone's 2WW is different and there are some great books, articles and blogs that you might like to read so that you know what you are thinking and feeling is absolutely, perfectly normal. See 'Two-Week Wait' for more information.

Sheila says: Waiting to hear how many eggs had fertilised after egg collection/retrieval was, for me, worse than the two-week wait. I remember being like a broody hen during this time – I felt as though I'd left a part of me behind and I hated the thought of my 'babies' being all alone in an incubator. I just wanted to be sitting next to the incubator watching and waiting until at least one was back inside me.

In Vitro Maturation – IVM

During a natural menstrual cycle, your ovaries contain many immature follicles and as you approach ovulation, one follicle matures and releases the mature egg – this is ovulation. With standard IVF, you are given hormones to stimulate your ovaries to produce a number of follicles each containing a mature egg.

With IVM, you are not given hormones because immature eggs are collected from the immature follicles in your ovaries before they mature, in the same way that mature eggs are collected/retrieved.

IVM may be suggested to you if:

- you are at risk from OHSS
- if you don't want to or can't take fertility drugs
- if you have PCOS
- male factor infertility is the cause for you being unable to get pregnant.

The below is not to scale and is purely an artistic impression of the egg collection/retrieval procedure.

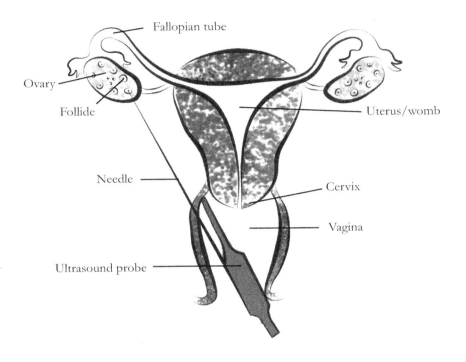

These immature eggs are matured in a dish in a special culture in the fertility clinic's laboratory for 24 to 48 hours. When the eggs are mature, they are fertilised with your partner's sperm or donor sperm, usually with ICSI.

The below is not to scale and is purely an artistic impression of ICSI.

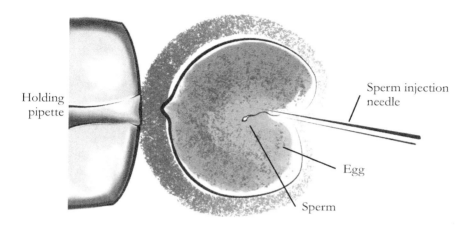

Holding pipette

Sperm injection needle

Egg

Sperm

As with IVF, the embryologist selects the best embryo to transfer back into your womb. To read more on the actual procedure see 'In Vitro Fertilisation'.

IVF Cycle

This is a round of IVF, including taking medications, having scans and blood tests, egg collection/retrieval, embryo transfer and finally ending with the pregnancy test. see 'In Vitro Fertilisation' for more information.

IVF Mild (Stimulation) – Mild IVF

The main difference between this and standard IVF is that less medication is used to stimulate your ovaries which means that it is kinder and safer to your body. Less eggs will be collected/retrieved than are collected in standard IVF. The risks of side effects from the medication is reduced so it may be suggested if you have experienced OHSS previously. If you have strong views about taking lots of medication or health concerns, this may be an option for you and you must discuss this with your clinic.

Once your eggs are collected/retrieved, the process is the same as standard IVF; your eggs are fertilised (hopefully) with your partners or a donor's sperm, embryos develop, the best embryo/s are transferred.

IVF Natural Cycle

This is another type of IVF but no down regulation or stimulation medication is given. You will have ultrasound scans of your ovaries to identify the dominant follicle and to check that your womb lining/endometrium is thickening. At the correct time, in the same way as in IVF, an egg is collected/retrieved from the dominant follicle in your ovary before you ovulate (you may be given medication to prevent spontaneous ovulation). The egg is then mixed with the sperm in the culture in the clinic's laboratory to wait for fertilisation to happen, or ICSI is carried out. Then the egg is checked for fertilisation and further development as with IVF. If the egg fertilises and develops, the embryo or blastocyst will be transferred into your womb on Day 2, Day 3 or Day 5.

It may be suggested to you as the better fertility treatment if:

- you previously had OHSS
- if you have responded poorly to previous IVF cycles
- if you have low ovarian reserve
- you don't want to take drugs that are used in standard IVF.

Because your follicles are not being stimulated, only one egg will mature so you only have this one chance and not the several that you hope to get with standard IVF.

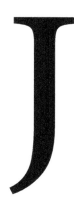

JOURNALING

The first IVF baby born in the US was born on 28 December 1981 and she was the 15th IVF baby to be born in the world.

Journaling

When you were a child did you keep a diary? A place where you wrote about your feelings, your plans, who you were going to marry, what job you were going to do, what made you angry…? If you are struggling to get pregnant, I'm sure you experience a whole range of emotions and feelings from one minute to the next, and this can leave you feeling exhausted and wrung out. If you are also having fertility treatment, this brings a whole new level of feelings and emotions. Regardless as to where you are on your fertility journey, you may find it useful to begin a fertility journal. Fertility coaches encourage you to do this as it is a useful tool; especially if you write and use it regularly, preferably every day. It may help to write at a certain time of the day or in a certain place at home – wherever and whenever, make it a habit.

How can it help you? Here are some reasons you may not have thought of:

- express your emotions without anyone judging you
- organise your thoughts
- record what you eat, drink and when
- record your energy levels
- record where you are in your menstrual cycle and what is happening
- record what your sleep pattern is like
- keep a track of fertility medications you are on, appointments, test results.

All the above may also help you to start seeing patterns – maybe after you eat a certain food you feel bloated, if you drink tea in the evening you struggle to get to sleep, meditating in the mornings makes your mood better all day, and so on. If you don't write these things down and read them you often miss what is very obvious about you and your body.

You can start your journal in a special notebook or you can buy a fertility journal straight away (there are many great ones available). Hopefully your journey to getting pregnant and welcoming your baby into your life won't be that long, but wouldn't it be amazing to show your journal to your child when they grow up. It would even be fantastic for you to read just how strong and persistent you were, because we forget a lot of what we went through as our memory fades or gets confused with our lives being so busy. After all, your fertility journey is part of your life and makes you who you are.

.

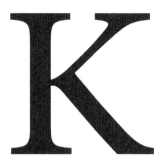

KARYOTYPE TEST to
KISSPEPTIN

Having sexual intercourse three to four times every week
gives most fertile couples the best chance of conceiving

Karyotype Test

Also called 'chromosome analysis'. This is a blood test and it looks at the structure, number and arrangement, or 'normalness', of all 46 chromosomes. If you are having problems getting pregnant or you have a history of miscarriages, you can have this test done to see if your infertility problems are due to an abnormality with your or your partners, chromosomes.

For example, you could have a condition called Turner syndrome, where you only have one X chromosome instead of two X chromosomes. A symptom of this syndrome is that you have not had any menstrual periods at all, which is known as primary amenorrhea. There is a variation of Turner syndrome called 'Turner mosaic' and this is when some cells in your body do not have the second X chromosome and symptoms of this are that you have premature ovarian failure at quite a young age, but you do have periods.

Kisspeptin

This is a natural hormone produced by the hypothalamus in your brain, and it may be used as an alternative 'trigger shot' to the more commonly used human chorionic gonadotropin (hCG), during ART cycles such as IVF. The trigger shot helps the follicles in your ovaries to mature the eggs and is administered about 36 hours prior to your egg collection/retrieval. For a number of women, especially those with PCOS, hCG causes OHSS, which is a potentially life-threatening condition – see 'Ovarian Hyperstimulation Syndrome' for more information.

The difference between kisspeptin and hCG is that kisspeptin causes the release of a hormone in your body which acts as a 'trigger' but hCG acts directly on the ovaries and can overstimulate them.

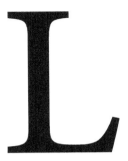

LAPAROSCOPY to
LYMPHOCYTE IMMUNISATION THERAPY

> 1,500 new sperm cells are 'born' every second.

Laparoscopy – LAP

This is a minor surgical procedure and enables a surgeon to see your uterus, Fallopian tubes and ovaries using a laparoscope, which is a thin, fibre optic telescope. It may be carried out to diagnose infertility or to treat a known fertility problem.

It is done under a general anaesthetic and you may be able to go home the same day or stay in hospital overnight. A small incision is made near your belly button and carbon dioxide gas (CO_2) is put into the abdomen to lift the abdominal wall and separate the abdominal organs so the reproductive organs can be seen easier. The laparoscope is then inserted and the doctor can see any abnormalities that may be causing you to have problems getting pregnant, such as:

- endometriosis
- pelvic adhesions
- ovarian cysts
- fibroids.

If abnormalities are found, the doctor can insert additional instruments through further small incisions (usually only two) and carry out a surgical procedure, such as removing a fibroid. All incisions are sewn up on completion of the procedure and covered with a dressing.

You may feel bloated from the CO_2 and will likely feel some pain, mostly in your shoulder tip because the CO_2 irritates the nerves under your diaphragm, for a day or two afterwards, and you should rest for at least 24 hours.

The below is not to scale and is an artistic impression of your reproductive system.

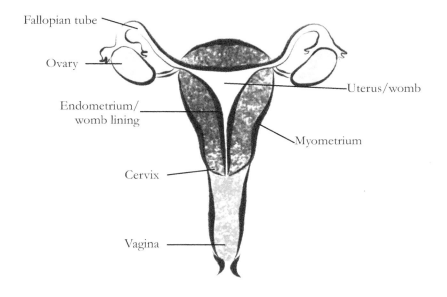

Laptops

Laptop use, especially if placed on a man's lap, may have a negative impact on his sperm count and sperm health because it raises the temperature of the testes/testicles. The reason for a man's testes being outside his body is because the temperature must be lower than his core body temperature by 2°F. A study showed that if a man had a laptop on his lap for an hour, the scrotal temperature increased by 5°F. Even positioning the laptop on top of a cushion or laptop pad doesn't help because, by sitting with the knees together, heat is trapped in the scrotal area and so raises the temperature of the scrotum.

It is still unknown if electromagnetic frequencies (EMF) from cellular devices such as mobile/cell phones and laptops affects the fertility of men and women. A more hidden issue regarding laptops is that both sexes are becoming more sedentary and long periods of inactivity can have a negative effect on fertility.

Laser Assisted Hatching – LAH

See 'Assisted Hatching' for more information.

Leptin

See 'Sleep' for more information.

Live Birth Rate - LMR

This is a statistic you will probably read on a fertility clinic website and its meaning varies depending on the country the clinic is in. An overview of this term is that it is the percentage of all ART cycles that result in the live birth of a baby. Multiple births are usually counted as one birth.

Long Protocol Cycle

This is the term used by your fertility clinic when you are starting an IVF cycle and the 'long' part refers to the length of time your hormones are switched off, known as 'down regulation' – see 'Down Regulation' for more information.

The down regulating medication is generally started on Day 21 of your menstrual cycle before the month when you are due to start treatment, and you take it for around two to three weeks. The medication is either an injection or a nasal spray and some side effects experienced are:

- mood swings
- hot flushes/flashes
- headaches.

These side effects are similar to side effects of the menopause and they go once you start your follicle-stimulating hormone (FSH) injections.

You may have an ultrasound scan or blood test to ensure that down regulation has occurred before you move onto taking the medication that stimulates your ovaries to produce more follicles and eggs.

Low Ovarian Reserve – LOR

Also known as 'diminished ovarian reserve' (DOR) and 'low functional ovarian reserve' (LFOR). You are born with all your eggs (around two million) and after puberty until your menopause, only one egg every month matures (unless you are already pregnant) and is released from your ovary ready to be fertilised. You would think then that you had a plentiful supply to last until your menopause, but approximately a thousand die every month, and by the age of 37 you only have about 25,000 eggs left.

Low ovarian reserve usually occurs when you are in your mid to late thirties; however, it can affect you if you are younger when it is known as 'premature ovarian failure'. It is believed that when you are 37/38 years old there is a faster decline of antral follicles or resting follicles – basically follicles with immature eggs in your ovaries that are awaiting their turn to start to mature. When you read statistics about it being more difficult to get pregnant after age

37/38 this is the reason why.

It's believed that a low ovarian reserve doesn't mean that the quality of your eggs is poorer as egg quality is age related. Therefore, having LOR may make it harder and it may take longer, but it is not impossible to get pregnant in your late 30s and early 40s

Antral follicle count (AFC) and anti-Müllerian hormone (AMH) are the two tests that are carried out to find out what your ovarian reserve is. See both these terms for more information.

Low Sperm Count

This is a common cause of male factor infertility and can make it more difficult to conceive naturally, although this can still happen. The medical term is oligozoospermia or oligospermia. The international guideline is that if there are fewer than 15 million sperm per millilitre of semen, this is considered a low count.

To find out what a man's sperm count is, he will have to produce a semen sample. A reliable result would be where the sample is sent off to a laboratory, and this way not only is the sperm counted but also how well they are moving can also be tested. There are home test kits that you can buy but they just test for the sperm count and nothing else. If the result is low then your doctor will probably suggest another test a few months later as the sperm count changes from day to day. Very often the cause for a low sperm count is unknown or your partner could have one of the following:

- a hormonal problem, such as hypogonadism

- a genetic problem

- varicoceles (enlarged veins in the testicles)

- blockage of the tubes that carry the sperm

- undescended testicles

- genital infection such as chlamydia or gonorrhoea.

Lifestyle habits can cause damage to sperm or even kill sperm, such as:

- excessive alcohol consumption

- using a sauna or spa which leads to overheating the testicles

- cigarette smoking

- drug use.

Even though your partner may have a low sperm count your doctor could advise that you keep trying naturally for the time being (if there are no other issues that could be causing you to be having problems getting pregnant), and to have sex every two to three days. They will also advise some lifestyle changes if appropriate, such as cutting down on alcohol, giving up smoking, healthy eating and exercising. If trying naturally for two years or more hasn't worked, your doctor may then discuss IVF or ICSI.

The below is not to scale and is an artistic impression of a sperm.

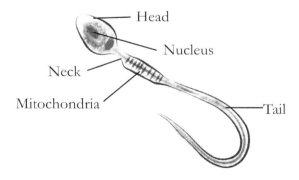

Lubricant

Seeking a vaginal lubricant whilst trying to get pregnant isn't uncommon, as the stress of having sex on schedule can lower your sex drive and therefore reduce the amount of naturally produced cervical mucus – see 'Cervical Mucus' for more information. Some fertility treatments, such as Clomid, may have a side effect of vaginal dryness (you have got to be kidding!). Also, some causes of infertility, such as hormonal imbalance and anovulation (you're not ovulating), can also reduce the amount of cervical mucus that you produce. Unknowingly, you may be affecting the quantity and quality of your cervical mucus if you do vaginal cleansing, such as douches; if you are concerned that you have an offensive vaginal odour speak to your doctor because if you have an infection, douching won't get rid of the infection.

Be very certain that, if you are going to use a lubricant, it is a sperm and vagina-friendly one. Some traditional lubricants that are used when you are not trying to get pregnant may damage sperm movement and DNA and can even kill sperm and/or affect your vaginal pH. Lubricants should not be used when providing a sperm/semen sample for testing or for fertility treatment such as IVF. It is also advised that you don't use saliva as a lubricant as it may affect the ability of the sperm to move. Therefore it's important to ask your fertility doctor or expert for advice and recommendations on fertility-friendly lubricants.

Luteal Phase Deficit/Defect – LPD

Your luteal phase (LP) occurs after ovulation up until your menstrual period, and is usually about 12 to 14 days long. During this phase, your ovaries make the hormone progesterone which tells your uterine lining/endometrium to thicken in preparation for a possible embryo to implant. An LPD occurs if your ovaries don't produce enough progesterone or your endometrium doesn't thicken in response to progesterone. It can be caused by a number of conditions, such as:

- short luteal phase
- PCOS
- extreme exercise
- too high or too low body mass index — see 'Body Mass Index' for more information
- thyroid disorders
- endometriosis.

If you have LPD you may notice that your periods are more frequent and shorter and you get spotting between periods. You may also experience early pregnancy loss and have trouble getting pregnant. To diagnose LPD your doctor will carry out blood tests to check your levels of follicle-stimulating hormone (FSH), luteinising hormone (LH) and progesterone and also do an ultrasound scan to measure the thickness of your endometrium.

The treatment is to correct any underlying medical condition and/or make lifestyle changes, and this is often all that is needed. Or your doctor may prescribe ovulation induction treatment.

Luteinised Unruptured Follicle Syndrome — LUFS

Also called 'trapped egg syndrome', this is when an egg matures fully or partially inside the follicle, the corpus luteum is created after the surge of luteinising hormone (LH), but the follicle doesn't rupture so the egg is not released. If you have LUFS, which incidentally is very rare, you will have all the signs that you are ovulating if you are looking out for the signs, so you will have a temperature rise due to the LH surge and your cervical mucus will change.

It is very difficult to diagnose and is done so by a series

of ultrasounds scans or by NaProTECHNOLOGY – see 'NaProTECHNOLOGY' for more information.

It is more likely to occur if you have:

- endometriosis
- PCOS – thought to be due to the ovary being tougher so would be harder for the follicle to rupture
- if you are taking nonsteroidal anti-inflammatory drugs (NSAIDs) as these drugs block normal prostaglandin activity that happens in the follicle
- taking the drug Clomid over multiple consecutive cycles.

If you have unexplained infertility it may be that LUFS is making it difficult for you to get pregnant.

Luteinising Hormone – LH

Also known as luteinizing hormone, lutropin, lutrophin and interstitial cell stimulating hormone. It is a hormone produced by the gonadotrophic cells in the pituitary gland, which is located in your brain. It is an important reproductive hormone in both you and in men. In you, LH has a different role depending on where you are in your menstrual cycle.

In weeks one to two of your menstrual cycle it stimulates the follicles in your ovaries to produce the sex hormone oestradiol – the main oestrogen/estrogen. Then, around Day 14 the LH levels surge causing the mature egg to be released from the follicle, otherwise known as ovulation.

For weeks three to four, what is left of the follicle forms a 'corpus luteum' and, if fertilisation occurs, the LH stimulates the corpus luteum to produce the hormone progesterone which is needed to support an early pregnancy.

In men, LH stimulates the production of testosterone in the testicles which in turn is important in sperm production.

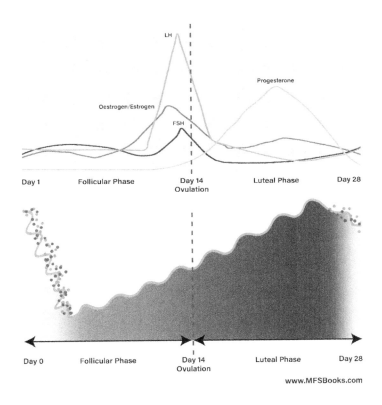

www.MFSBooks.com

Luteinising Hormone (LH) Surge

The level of LH is low throughout your menstrual cycle until the developing follicle in your ovary reaches a certain size which causes the amount of oestrogen to reach a certain level. The oestrogen level tells the pituitary gland to release a very high amount or a surge of LH. It is this surge that brings about ovulation, release of the egg from the follicle 24 to 36 hour later. After ovulation your LH levels drop. See above diagram.

You can find out when you get your LH surge by using ovulation predictor kits (OPKs) or by recording and charting your basal body temperature (BBT) – see 'Basal Body Temperature Charting'.

Lymphocyte Immunisation Therapy – LIT

This is a treatment that your doctor may suggest if you have had miscarriages or implantation failures during IVF, and the cause is believed to be due to you not accepting the embryo because your body thinks it's a foreign body and you make antibodies to fight it.

This is a controversial treatment and not all fertility experts believe that it helps and that it should be used.

LIT is where white blood cells from the father-to-be or a donor are injected into the skin of your forearm to help your immune system to recognise and accept the embryo. There are no side effects to you but you may experience a rash or redness at the injection site.

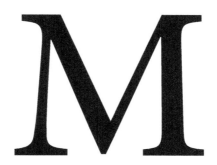

MAGNETIC-ACTIVATED CELL SORTING to
MORULA

On average, it takes almost four-and-a-half years to conceive with IVF. (HFEA)

Magnetic-Activated Cell Sorting – MACS

This is a technique used for sorting out sperm in a semen sample that has damaged DNA. For a fertilised egg to develop into an embryo then a blastocyst, the sperm that fertilised the egg needs to be of a good quality. A high amount of DNA damage in the sperm will affect the development of the embryo and lead to it not developing normally or result in an early miscarriage.

DNA damage will eventually cause the sperm to die and this type of damage cannot be identified during the normal semen analysis that looks at the morphology (appearance) and motility (movement) of sperm; see both these terms for more information. The major causes of sperm DNA damage are:

- oxidative stress caused by, for example, cigarette smoking
- drug use
- environmental pollutants
- inflammatory infection
- getting older.

The MACS process to remove the damaged and dying sperm is to wash the sample, then microscopic magnetic balls are placed into this sample. The balls stick to the sperm that have DNA damage. A magnetic field attracts the sperm with the beads and they are removed before the rest of the sperm are used for fertility treatment, such as IVF or ICSI.

Male Factor Infertility – MF

Refers to a man's inability to make you pregnant when you are fertile. The World Health Organisation (WHO) defines it as 'the presence of more than one abnormality in the semen analysis or the presence of inadequate sexual or ejaculatory function'.

It used to be thought that only we women were infertile but now it is known that of all infertility cases, a third are due to male factor infertility. It is estimated that 1 in 20 men has some sort of infertility problem. In most cases there are no signs or symptoms of infertility, with intercourse, erection and ejaculation usually happening without any difficulty.

It is generally caused by either problems that affect sperm production or sperm moving from where they are made to where they leave his body.

1. Sperm production

About two-thirds of infertile men have a problem with making sperm – either they don't make enough, so have a low sperm count, or the sperm that are produced have something wrong with them; this is known as 'morphology' and 'motility'. Both of these terms are explained further in this book. Production problems can be due to:

- congenital (from birth) problems with his testicles/testes

- undescended testicles at birth

- imbalances of reproductive hormones, such as testosterone, follicle-stimulating hormone (FSH) and luteinising hormone (LH)

- infections

- varicoceles (varicose veins of the testicles)

- exposure to environmental chemicals/toxins, such as smoking or alcohol
- certain medicines
- cancer treatment.

Some of these issues can be overcome, which means that sperm numbers can be increased and the condition of the sperm themselves can be corrected – remember a man is continually making new sperm. It is important that he sees a fertility specialist, reproductive endocrinologist or reproductive urologist.

2. Sperm moving from where they are made to where they need to be

About one in five infertile men have a problem with getting sperm from where it is made to where it needs to be to make a baby. The problems are blockages or obstructions in the tubes that carry sperm from the testicles to the penis and can be caused by:

- previous surgery such as a vasectomy
- infection that hasn't been treated or was treated too late
- congenital abnormalities of the tubes.

These issues may be able to be corrected with reconstructive surgery or obtaining the sperm directly from the testicles for IVF or ICSI.

As with women, men can also have unexplained infertility.

It often comes as a huge shock when a man finds out he has fertility issues – he feels the same emotions that we feel when it's female factor; he'll be angry with himself, blame himself, be jealous of other men, depressed, won't want to speak about it to anyone – the feelings are endless. Quite often when the issue is male factor the woman will take the blame when they are telling others, to 'protect' him. There isn't as much support for men as there is for you and often men find it even harder than us to share how they are feeling.

But it is equally important that he too has support from somewhere and counselling or a support group at a clinic, for example, may be worth looking into.

> **Sheila says: Some Facebook support groups and fertility forums are getting much better at offering support for men, so if your partner isn't keen to go to an actual support group (though he's unlikely to be the only man), he may find online support better than nothing. Many men who are dealing with or have dealt with male factor infertility are blogging, too, so this may also be of help.**

The below is not to scale and is an artistic impression of a sperm.

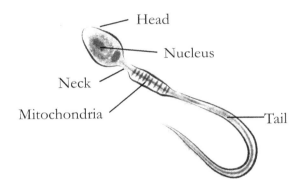

Male Hormone Profile Test

This is a blood test to check the hormone levels that are concerned with fertility in men. The hormones tested are:

- luteinising hormone (LH) and follicle-stimulating hormone (FSH), produced by the pituitary gland. Low levels of either hormone can cause low or no sperm production

- thyroid stimulating hormone (TSH), T3 and T4 – these are tested to diagnose thyroid disorders and to monitor hypothyroidism and hyperthyroidism, as hypothyroidism will result in a low sperm count and sperm defects, and hyperthyroidism may damage sperm

- testosterone - low levels of this male sex hormone cause low sperm count

- sex hormone binding globulin (SHBG) – this evaluates the male sex hormones such as testosterone

- prolactin levels – high levels affect the functionality of the testicles and can cause decreased testosterone levels or abnormal sperm leading to infertility.

All these terms are explained further in this book.

Metformin

This is a drug usually given to people with diabetes to control their insulin levels. If you have PCOS your doctor may prescribe you metformin either with or without Clomid, and also possibly during IVF.

The reason for prescribing you this drug is because often, if you have PCOS, you are also insulin resistant, though this isn't the case for everyone – see 'Polycystic Ovarian/Ovary Syndrome' for more information. It is not clear how metformin improves fertility but there appears to be a connection between insulin and the reproductive hormones; increased insulin levels lead to increased androgen hormone levels. Metformin lowers excess levels of insulin which regulates the reproductive hormones and brings about ovulation.

As with a number of areas of fertility treatment, there are different opinions as to whether Metformin is effective if you have PCOS and are insulin resistance. Seek medical advice if you want to find out more.

Methylenetetrahydrofolate Reductase – MTHFR

If you can say this term you're a better person than I am! All of us have the same set of genes and it is the variations in these genes that make each of us unique. The MTHFR gene helps us to metabolise (breakdown and use) folate, which is a water-soluble B vitamin (Vitamin B9) and is needed by our bodies to make DNA and for cells to divide. Most of us aren't aware that folate and folic acid are not the same – folate is found naturally in food but folic acid is a man-made synthetic used in supplements and is inactive, meaning it needs to be broken down by your body many times before it is absorbed.

Each of us have around 34 MTHFR genes but two of them are where most of the research is focused, and they are C677 and A1298. Like all of our genes, the MTHFR gene can be changed or mutated and this mutation can cause some chronic illnesses, such as cardiovascular disease and blood clotting. MTHFR mutation has also been linked to miscarriage because the mutation may make it difficult to sustain a pregnancy. This is due to the MTHFR gene only allowing 30-50% of the folate to be used by your body.

When you are trying to get pregnant it is advised that you take a prenatal supplement and most of these contain folic acid. The reason for this is because folic acid is vital for early development of a baby and prevents neural tube defects such as spina bifida. If you do not have MTHFR issues folic acid certainly helps. However, if you have a mutation and you take a folic acid supplement, natural folate will not be able to be absorbed by the cells because the folic acid is being converted first. If cells are not getting folate, the growing baby is being deprived of folate which affects its development and growth.

Micro-epididymal Sperm Aspiration – MESA

In some men's semen there are no sperm because of a blocked vas deferens or because they were born without any vasa deferentia. The vasa deferentia are two tiny tubes that carry sperm from the testicles/testes to the end of the penis. MESA is a surgical procedure usually carried out under general anaesthetic that removes sperm surgically from the epididymis. A small cut is made in the scrotum and with the aid of a microscope, the tubules of the epididymis are located and the sperm are removed.

With this procedure a large number of sperm can be removed that can be frozen and used in future ART cycles, such as ICSI – see 'Intracytoplasmic Sperm Injection' for more information.

The below is not to scale and is an artistic impression of the male reproductive system.

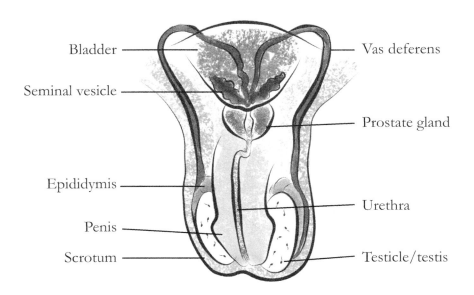

Micromanipulation

This is a term used for advanced techniques that use powerful microscopes and specialised equipment in ART. Using these techniques may improve the chances of pregnancy when the male partner only produces a small number of sperm, and one such technique is ICSI – see 'Intracytoplasmic Sperm Injection' for more information.

Mild or Minimal Stimulation In Vitro Fertilisation (IVF)

See 'IVF Mild Stimulation' for more information.

Miscarriage

This is the loss of your baby before 24 weeks of pregnancy. If you miscarry in the first 12 weeks it is called an 'early miscarriage' and if your loss is between 12 and 24 weeks, it's called a 'late miscarriage'. The main symptoms are vaginal bleeding or spotting with or without abdominal pain or cramping. Sometimes there are no obvious signs – this is called a 'missed miscarriage'; see this term for more information.

It is estimated that in the UK, miscarriages occur in one in four recognised pregnancies with 85% of those occurring in the first 12 weeks. As you get older you are more likely to have a miscarriage than someone who is younger; if you are under 30, you have a 1 in 10 chance of miscarrying, and if you are over 45, you have a 5 in 10 chance of having a miscarriage.

The cause of early miscarriages is still unknown but it is thought to be due to genetic or chromosomal problem in the developing baby.

If you have symptoms your miscarriage is usually confirmed by an ultrasound scan. During a routine scan if you have had no symptoms, this may be when you find out you have miscarried your baby.

If you have three or more miscarriages in a row, doctors call this 'recurrent miscarriage'. You should be referred to a gynaecologist so that you can have tests and investigations to find out why. However, in about half of the cases of recurrent miscarriage the doctor cannot find a reason, which is extremely upsetting and frustrating for you. Even if no reason is found, it may still mean that you have a chance of a successful pregnancy the next time. Although there are some conditions that cause recurrent miscarriage, they are uncommon but may include:

- anti-phospholipid syndrome (APS) – also known as sticky blood syndrome or Hughes syndrome – see APS for more information

- Thrombophilia – see this term for more information

- genetic problems

- problems with your womb or cervix

- bacterial vaginosis – see this term for more information

- hormone problems

- polycystic ovaries – see this term for more information.

Stress, depression and shock do not cause you to have a miscarriage.

There are some things you can do to reduce your risk of having a miscarriage, such as stopping smoking, not drinking alcohol or taking illegal drugs when pregnant, and limiting your caffeine intake.

Experiencing a miscarriage can be devastating and extremely heart breaking regardless of how early it happens. You may feel shock, anger, jealousy, empty and lonely – all these are common feelings. Everyone is different but you do need to give yourself time to grieve for your baby. If you have a partner they will also need time to come to terms with your loss, as may other family members.

It is sadly quite common to find that other people, and they can be close family and friends, don't understand how devastated you are after a miscarriage, and they say thoughtless things like 'You can get pregnant again' or 'It was meant to be'. This is terribly hurtful as you wanted this baby and no, it wasn't meant to happen to this baby. You may find it helps instead to talk about it especially to someone you know who has also had a miscarriage – you may be surprised how many people you know have also had a miscarriage when you tell them, as a lot of people keep it to themselves. Alternatively, there are support groups, Facebook groups and online forums if you prefer to 'talk' to someone you don't know.

It is nothing to be ashamed of as you have done nothing wrong and it definitely is not your fault. There is no reason why you shouldn't try again to get pregnant straight away – you are advised not to because it may be difficult to know your dates if you do get pregnant straight away again.

You may find that having a service to remember your baby helps with your grieving and gives you closure regardless of how many weeks pregnant you were.

Sheila says: I had a miscarriage after our second ICSI cycle at six weeks. I have never experienced such two extremes of emotions in a heartbeat – one moment we were expecting our baby because the blood test had said so, and then a heartbeat later, the scan showed that there was no baby any more. Just like that. Given such a precious gift for it to be snatched away. How do you get over this? We all cope in different ways and often we think we're coping when we're really not. I found out several years after the miscarriage that I had suffered post-traumatic stress disorder (PTSD). This isn't uncommon at all. It is really important to talk to either a professional or someone at a support group if you are feeling anxiety, depression and distress.

Missed Miscarriage – MM

Also called 'delayed miscarriage' or 'silent miscarriage', this is when your baby has died or has not developed as expected, but your body has not let him or her go. The scan will show a pregnancy sac with your baby (even if it's an embryo, it's still your baby), but there is no heartbeat and your baby will probably be smaller than expected. You probably still feel pregnant and if you did a pregnancy test it would be positive and this is because the pregnancy hormone levels are still high.

See 'Miscarriage' above for more information, especially on coping after a miscarriage.

Your options are to wait for nature to take its course, taking tablets or pessaries to bring about the miscarriage or surgery – see 'Dilation & Evacuation' for more information.

Morula

This is the medical term for a Day 3 or Day 4 fertilised egg but generally everyone calls it an 'embryo' or 'emby'. It is now a cluster of around 12-30 cells and resembles a mulberry (morula is Latin for mulberry).

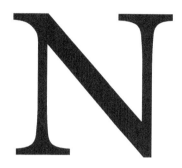

NAPRO TECHNOLOGY

to

NON-MOTILE SPERM

An egg is not able to move – it moves from the ovary to the Fallopian tube by being wafted by hair-like projections called cilia.

NaProTECHNOLOGY – NPT

This brand name stands for 'Natural Procreative Technology' and has been around since the early 1990s. It came about following the Catholic Church, in 1968, asking scientists and medical professionals to develop a way that a married couple could manage the size of their family based on an understanding of the body's natural rhythms. A gynaecologist in the US, Dr Tom Hilgers, studied thousands of women's menstrual cycle charts to find out when they were and weren't fertile and, in doing so, he also found that the charts provided useful information about the women's gynaecological health. This approach is used for infertility as well as recurrent miscarriage. I'm not endorsing the brand and have no connection with the company.

National Institute for Health and Care Excellence (UK only) – NICE

This is only relevant to the UK and is a Non-Departmental Public Body as set out in the Health and Social Care Act 2012. It provides national guidance and advice to improve health and social care and it operates independently of the government. The way NICE was established in legislation means that its guidance is officially England-only. However, it has agreements to provide certain NICE products and services to Wales, Scotland and Northern Ireland.

The NICE guidelines are, that where infertility is concerned, everyone should be offered up to three cycles of IVF (providing certain criteria are met), but unfortunately this is rarely the case. It is commonly termed the 'Post Code Lottery' and you need to contact your local Clinical Commissioning Group, or CCG.

Natural Cycle IVF – NC IVF

See 'IVF Natural Cycle' for more information.

Natural Killer Cells – NKC

There are NKCs in your blood and they occur naturally as part of your immune system. Their role is to recognise and 'kill' cells (hence their name), which should not be in your body, such as infections, viruses and cancers. In your uterus you have uterine natural killer (uNK) cells, but their function is not clearly understood as it is a difficult area to study. One possible function of uNK cells that some experts believe they have, is to get rid of inflammatory stressed cells in the endometrium (womb lining) to make space for the embryo to implant. Another possible function is that when the embryo implants, the placenta blood cells (which are made by the developing embryo) have to dig into the womb lining and make contact with your blood cells in order for your blood to nourish your baby, and the uNK cells help this to happen.

Some fertility experts however believe that the uNK cells recognise the embryo as a foreign body and attack it, causing recurrent miscarriages and repeated implantation failures. Others don't believe this is the case.

Those experts who believe there is a connection between uNK cells and miscarriage/implantation failure may offer tests that measure your uNK cells by carrying out a blood test and/or by doing an endometrial biopsy – see 'Endometrial Biopsy' for more information. There are some very highly regarded UK fertility experts who disagree with these tests being carried out for recurrent miscarriage/implantation failure for two reasons:

1. There is no globally accepted measurement range for uNK cells testing which means any results are difficult to interpret

2. As there is no clear link between blood and uterine NK cells testing your blood for NK cells may not be worth doing.

The treatment that is offered at certain fertility clinics is reproductive immune therapy, such as intravenous immunoglobulin or IVIg; see this term in this book for more information. As this is a very grey area and in most countries the treatment offered isn't regulated (in the UK, the HFEA doesn't support the treatment), it is very important you are cautious and do your research and seek a second opinion if appropriate.

Natural Killer Cell Assay – NK Assay

This is a test to check the sensitivity of the NK cells to foreign tissue and also the killing power of the NK cells. This test may be suggested to you by your doctor. There are two parts to the test:

1. To analyse the percentage of target cells that are killed by the NK cells

2. To find out if, by adding the different treatment options, e.g. IVIg, the killing powers of the NK cells is reduced or not, thus determining which is the best treatment.

Necrozoospermia

Also called 'necrospermia', this is when the sperm in a fresh semen sample are dead. 'Complete necrozoospermia' is very rare and is when all the sperm are dead. 'Incomplete necroszoospermia' is when less than 45% but more than 5% of the sperm in the sample are alive. Usually a man will not know he has necrozoospermia until he has a semen sample tested. Very often, when the result indicates necroszoospermia, it is a mistake and the reasons for this are:

- a non-fertility friendly lubricant was used to help collect the sample and these can kill sperm
- the container used to collect the sample was dirty or contaminated
- the sperm sample was collected in a condom during intercourse and latex can kill sperm.

Therefore, if your male partner receives a diagnosis of necrozoospermia your doctor will ask him to produce another sample.

The cause of necrozoospermia is often unknown because it is so rare but some suggestions are:

- infection in the reproductive tract
- testicular problems
- hormonal causes
- abnormally high body temperature in the scrotum
- anti-sperm antibodies
- exposure to toxins
- advanced age.

Where the cause is found, treatment is advised where possible - for example, antibiotics if the cause is due to an infection. If no cause is found for complete necrozoospermia, a surgical procedure called testicular sperm extraction or TESE – see this term for more information, will extract testicular tissue that contains immature, live sperm cells. In order to get pregnant, you would need to use

ICSI. Alternatively, pregnancy may only be achieved with donor sperm.

The below is not to scale and is an artistic impression of a sperm.

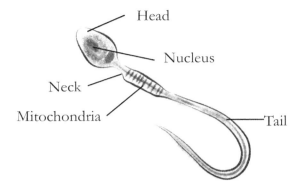

Next Generation Sequencing – NGS

This is a comprehensive chromosome testing technique to help fertility specialists to better select which embryo is more likely to implant in your womb and become a healthy baby. It is a similar test to pre-implantation genetic testing for aneuploidy or PGT-A, but NGS tests all 23 pairs of chromosomes and looks at the DNA in more detail and can detect when an embryo has cells that are not chromosomally correct (known as 'mosaicism').

Non-motile sperm

These are sperm that are not moving in a semen sample – they are not dead but for some reason they cannot move. In the semen analysis report, this may be indicated by 'IM' or 'immotile' or 'grade d'. Causes could be:

- genetic
- environmental
- poor nutrition
- heat exposure.

See 'Sperm Motility' for more information.

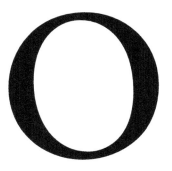

OBSTETRICIAN/GYNAECOLOGIST

to

OXIDATIVE STRESS

80% of ovulation problems in women are caused by polycystic ovaries. (HFEA)

Obstetrician/Gynaecologist – OB/GYN

This is a doctor who has completed their medical training and has further studied to specialise in female reproductive health and pregnancy. The obstetrician focuses on the care of the pregnant woman, the unborn baby, labour, delivery and the immediate period following childbirth. The gynaecologist focuses on any problems concerned with your reproductive organs: uterus/womb, Fallopian tubes, ovaries, cervix and vagina. They may also treat bowel, bladder and urinary system problems as they are closely related to your reproductive organs.

The below is not to scale and is an artistic impression of your reproductive system.

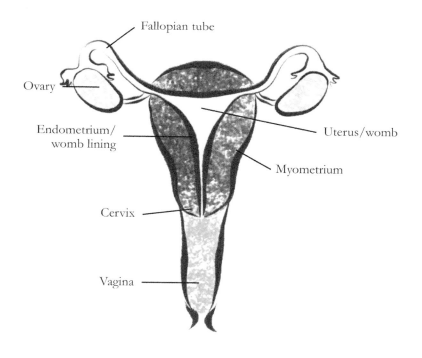

Oestradiol/Oestrogen/Oestriol

Also called estradiol, estrogen and estriol and are often known collectively as oestrogens, although oestrogen is a separate hormone in its own right.

Oestradiol is a steroid hormone made from cholesterol and is the strongest of these three naturally produced oestrogens. This hormone has many functions though its main ones are to mature and maintain your reproductive system. During your menstrual cycle, it causes an egg to mature and be released (ovulation), as well as thickening the uterine lining to receive a fertilised egg.

Oestrogen is produced by the ovaries and, like oestradiol, is responsible for the development of your reproductive system from puberty and regulating your menstrual cycle. When the follicles in your ovaries begin to mature they produce oestrogen, which results in ovulation. Therefore, if you are not producing enough oestrogen you will not ovulate.

Oestriol is also a steroid and is much weaker than the other two when you are not pregnant – in fact, levels are almost undetectable. During pregnancy the levels are much higher. It is made by the placenta from a chemical that comes from the baby's adrenal gland.

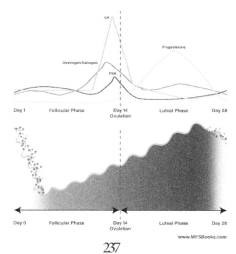

Oligoasthenoteratozoospermia – OAT

This is a condition where a man has a combination of three issues with his sperm;

- a low sperm count (oligozoospermia – see this term or 'Sperm' for more information)
- a low number of sperm with poor movement or motility (asthenozoospermia – see this term for more information)
- abnormal sperm shape or morphology (teratozoospermia – see this term for more information).

It is a common cause of male factor infertility and the chances of a natural pregnancy are quite low but not impossible. However, using ART will increase your chances.

The causes are:

- genetic
- lifestyle
- the testicles' inability to produce sperm of sufficient quantity or quality
- testicular and ejaculatory dysfunction.

Such genetic factors are DNA damage in sperm cells, defects in the Y chromosome and genetic disorders.

Most lifestyle habits and conditions that directly affect the sperm can be changed and therefore improve the chances of achieving a pregnancy. Such habits/conditions are: smoking, alcohol consumption, obesity, overheating the testicles and medications used to treat conditions unrelated to fertility, such as rheumatoid arthritis and bladder infections.

Testicular factors that affect the quantity and quality of sperm produced could be previous infections (syphilis, mumps, malaria), testicular trauma, variocele (varicose veins in the scrotum) and older age. Some can be treated but others can't.

Testicular and ejaculatory dysfunction are any conditions that affect a man's ability to ejaculate or which obstructs the flow of semen in the genital tract. Some conditions are obstruction of the vas deferens (narrow tubes in the testicles), inflammation of the prostate gland, hypospadias (a congenital defect where the opening of the urethra is not on the head of the penis) and erectile dysfunction.

Because there are different causes or sometimes no cause is found, the treatment will vary depending on the cause.

The below is not to scale and is an artistic impression of a sperm.

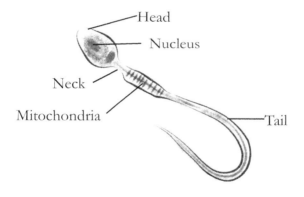

Oligoovulation

This is when you have irregular menstrual periods – less than eight a year or very long periods of more than 50 days. Because your periods are irregular it means that you ovulate irregularly, therefore this could be a cause of infertility. To diagnose oligoovulation you would have blood tests/blood work carried out on certain days of your period to measure the levels of certain hormones. You would also have a scan done of your ovaries to check follicle development, which would indicate if your ovaries are working as they should.

It can be caused by excess stress, eating disorders and tumours. Irregular periods are a common sign of polycystic ovary/ovarian syndrome or PCOS – see this term for more information.

Oligozoospermia/Oligospermia

This is a where a man has a low sperm count; fewer than 15 million sperm per millilitre of semen is the international guideline. See 'Sperm' for more information.

Oocyte

This is an immature egg cell that is produced in a follicle in your ovary. During your menstrual cycle, one oocyte usually matures due to hormones and becomes a mature egg. During IVF, ICSI and their variations, a number of oocytes will (hopefully) become mature eggs that are surgically collected/retrieved. Immature eggs are collected during in vitro maturation (IVM) – see this term for more information.

Ovarian Drilling

This is a procedure that your doctor may advise if you have PCOS – see 'Polycystic Ovary/Ovarian Syndrome' for more information. With PCOS, sometimes your ovaries have a thick outer surface and this can affect ovulation and therefore your ability to get pregnant. What ovarian drilling does is to break through this thick outer layer and destroys small portions of it. Ovarian drilling decreases testosterone production which means that you will likely ovulate more regularly.

You will have probably gone through all the other treatments for PCOS first because ovarian drilling is a surgical procedure. It is carried out under general anaesthetic as an outpatient and your recovery time is quite quick. This is what will happen during ovarian drilling:

A small incision is made below your belly button and the surgeon inserts a small tube into your abdomen and fills it with carbon dioxide (CO_2) gas. This helps to move your abdomen away from your ovaries so the surgeon can reach them easier. A thin telescope with a camera attached called a laparoscope is then inserted into your abdomen. Using the camera as a guide, the surgeon inserts special tools and uses an electric current to make very small holes on your ovaries.

If after this procedure your periods become regular, your chances of getting pregnant are good. But even if they don't become regular, you may still be able to get pregnant with the help of fertility drugs.

For some, the benefits are short lived as PCOS symptoms and fertility problems may return over time and your periods could become irregular again. You need to discuss ovarian drilling fully with your doctor in order to be able to decide if this procedure is best for you.

Ovarian Hyperstimulation Syndrome – OHSS

This is a medical condition that you may experience if you take fertility medication to stimulate your ovaries to mature more eggs when undergoing IVF, ovulation induction (OI) or IUI. The symptoms of OHSS often begin within seven to ten days after doing the 'trigger shot' to stimulate ovulation. Symptoms range from mild to severe and may worsen if it's not treated.

Mild to moderate symptoms include:

- abdominal pain
- abdominal bloating
- nausea
- vomiting
- diarrhoea
- tenderness in the area over your ovaries
- a sudden increase in weight of more than 3 kg/6.6 pounds.

With mild OHSS the symptoms may go away after a week.

Severe OHSS symptoms include:

- rapid weight gain of 15-20 kgs/33-44 pounds in five to ten days
- severe abdominal pain
- nausea and vomiting
- a decrease in the amount you pee
- shortness of breath and tightness
- enlarged abdomen.

Severe OHSS can lead to serious illness and death, though this is very rare, so any signs, even if mild, should be reported to your fertility doctor immediately.

The actual cause is unknown but it is related to high levels of the hormone human chorionic gonadotropin (hCG) being introduced to your body as the 'trigger shot' to mature your eggs for egg collection. The blood vessels in the ovaries react abnormally to the hCG and fluid begins to leak out. This fluid swells your ovaries and sometimes large amounts spill into your abdomen.

You are more at risk of OHSS if you have:

- polycystic ovary/ovarian syndrome (PCOS)
- are under 30 years old
- have a large number of follicles and rapidly rising oestrogen levels
- have a low body weight.

If you have symptoms it is likely that after egg collection/retrieval, you will be advised to freeze all your embryos and then, in a couple of months' time have one of the frozen embryos thawed then transferred. This is because if you do have an embryo or blastocyst transferred straight away and you get pregnant, the OHSS will worsen because your body will produce hCG naturally.

Ovarian Monitoring

This refers to closely observing you when you are undergoing fertility treatment such as IVF. This is because you will be taking hormones to stimulate your ovaries to mature more follicles and to produce as many eggs as possible.

During the time you are taking the nasal spray or doing injections, you will have regular (how regular depends on your clinic) ultrasound scans only or scans and blood tests. The scans are usually vaginal scans with a 'wand' which give a better view of your womb and how your womb lining is developing. The blood test is to check the level of the hormone oestradiol/estradiol, which is necessary to know when is the best time for you to do the 'trigger shot' to bring about ovulation, and also to identify if you are at risk from developing OHSS – see explanation above. Do ask questions if you don't understand any results – no question is ever a silly one.

When the leading follicle (that's the biggest one), reaches a diameter of 18 mm or over, and the lining of your womb is at least 8 mm thick and the oestradiol level is within normal limits, you will be told to do the 'trigger shot/injection'. The trigger injection is the hormone human chorionic gonadotropin (hCG) and this starts the process of maturing the eggs. You usually do it in the late evening and your egg collection/retrieval is 36 hours later.

Sheila says: When all this ovarian monitoring is going on, you will probably be very emotional and will be more obsessed than usual with your ovaries and womb. This is totally understandable and perfectly normal because everything is now riding on how many follicles are developing and how thick your womb lining is becoming. You will find yourself hanging onto every word the nurses and doctors are saying, and it is very easy to feel down if things are not going according to plan. If you are on forums and have some cycle buddies (women who are going through fertility treatment and IVF at the same time as you), it is very upsetting and discouraging if everyone else seems to be doing better than you are. Fertility forums certainly have their place but remember that everyone is different, there is no one reason for infertility and just because you don't have as many follicles as someone else, it doesn't mean to say this cycle won't work. Hard though it is, try to remain positive and be kind to yourself.

Ovarian Reserve

This is the term used by fertility experts regarding the potential number of immature eggs in your ovaries. As you age this number declines along with egg quality. Your genetics strongly influence your initial ovarian reserve. Also, high androgen (male hormone) levels during your development when you were inside your mother's womb have an unfavourable effect on establishing your ovarian reserve.

Your ovarian reserve is important in predicting how you will respond to the drugs used to stimulate your ovaries during ART such as IVF. There are tests to determine your ovarian reserve whether you are undergoing fertility treatment or you just want to know what yours is;

- two blood tests, one to measure follicle-stimulating hormone (FSH) on Day 3 of your menstrual cycle and a second to measure your level of anti-Müllerian hormone (AMH)
- the other test is an ultrasound scan of the antral follicles in your ovaries.

See 'anti-Müllerian hormone' and 'Antral Follicle Count' for more information.

Ovarian Stimulation – OS

This is the second stage of fertility treatments such as IVF, and the goal is to collect or retrieve as many mature eggs from the follicles in your ovaries as possible, to improve your chances of getting pregnant and becoming a parent. Before you start this stage, you will have blood tests so that your doctor knows the baseline levels of certain hormones in your body. This ensures your treatment regime is specific to you.

To produce as many mature eggs as possible, you will inject medication of two key hormones, namely follicle-stimulating hormone (FSH) and luteinising hormone (LH) for 8-14 days. During this time, you will have vaginal scans to measure the number and size of the follicles, and some clinics also do blood tests to measure the levels of the hormones in your blood. This means that you will be going to your fertility clinic regularly for a couple of weeks when you are probably also working – this can be very stressful and your clinic will understand this.

Because there is a lot to remember and it's a stressful period, if you are unsure as to what medication you should be taking and when (this is very easily done), it is really important that you call your clinic because if there is a problem it could affect the outcome of this IVF cycle. See also 'Ovarian Monitoring' for more information.

Ovary/Ovaries

Your ovaries are the most important part of your reproductive system and each ovary is about the size of an almond. They are on opposite sides of your uterus in the pelvic cavity and are attached to the uterus by a ligament. The open ends of your Fallopian tubes lie next to the ovaries but are not actually connected.

Their function is to produce the reproductive hormones oestrogen/estrogen and progesterone, and also to release an egg, known as 'ovulation', every month during your menstrual cycle for fertilisation. Your ovaries are controlled by gonadotropin-releasing hormone (GnRH), which is released by nerve cells in the hypothalamus in your brain and send messages to your pituitary gland to produce luteinising hormone (LH) and follicle-stimulating hormone (FSH) to control your menstrual cycle.

The below is not to scale and is an artistic impression of your reproductive system.

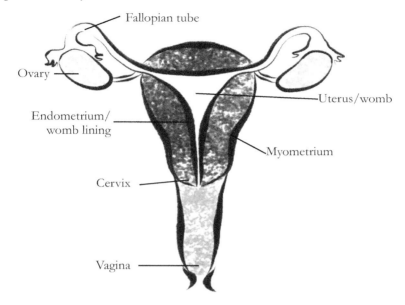

Overweight

Being overweight could affect your chances of getting pregnant and/or lengthening the time it takes for you to get pregnant. A man's fertility may also be affected if he is overweight too. See the term 'Body Mass Index' if you want to work out if you are overweight or not.

If you are overweight or obese, this can cause an imbalance in your hormones which could affect your fertility, because hormones have to be very finely balanced in order for you to get pregnant; a common hormonal condition that affects your weight is PCOS. You are also twice as likely to have a miscarriage than a woman who is of a healthy weight.

Once pregnant, you are more at risk of medical conditions, such as pre-eclampsia, pregnancy-related diabetes and high blood pressure.

Even your baby is more at risk of becoming an overweight child.

If a man is overweight/obese this could reduce his sperm count and concentration, reduce the ability of his sperm to move (motility) and negatively affect the shape of his sperm (morphology). It can also cause hormonal changes, especially lowering his levels of testosterone that could reduce his fertility and his interest in sex. He may also have problems getting an erection.

If being overweight/obese is a result of your lifestyles, changing your diet to a healthy one and exercising sensibly will help improve both your fertility and your likelihood of getting pregnant naturally. If it is a result of a medical condition, you must seek the advice of your doctor.

Ovulation

This is when a mature follicle that has been developing in your ovary releases a mature egg. If all the hormones concerned with fertility are being produced in the right amounts at the correct times during your menstrual cycle, and there are no other problems, then ovulation will occur. Usually only one follicle and egg mature but in some women two will mature and two eggs will be released during ovulation, and this could result in non-identical twins.

If your cycles are regular, ovulation usually happens approximately 12 to 16 days before your next period starts. Your body produces higher levels of oestrogen as you get nearer to ovulation and these high levels bring about a sudden surge of luteinising hormone (LH), produced in the pituitary gland. About 24 to 36 hours after this surge, ovulation occurs. You may feel a twinge in the area of your ovaries but if you don't, this doesn't mean you are not ovulating. There are no physical signs of ovulation.

Once the egg pops out of the follicle, tiny hair-like projections called cilia move it towards the opening of the Fallopian tube where, if there are sperm nearby, fertilisation may occur. The egg only lives for 24 hours after ovulation so timings are really crucial. If it isn't fertilised, hormone levels drop and your womb lining is shed, along with the egg.

See 'Follicle' for more information.

The below is not to scale and is an artistic impression of ovulation.

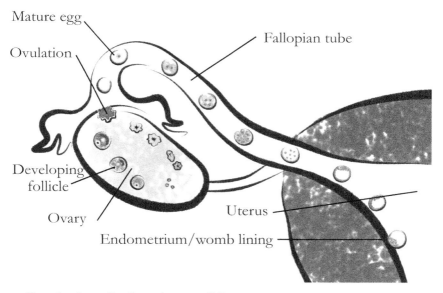

Mature egg

Ovulation

Fallopian tube

Developing follicle

Ovary

Uterus

Endometrium/womb lining

Ovulation Induction – OI

This is a fertility treatment that you may have if you do not ovulate (naturally develop and release an egg from one of your ovaries). This is usually indicated by irregular or absent periods. The common causes are:

- PCOS

- incorrect hormone levels

- stress

- weight fluctuations.

OI is where medication is taken at the beginning of your menstrual cycle, as a tablet or as an injection, to stimulate egg development in the follicles.

The commonly used medicine is called clomiphene citrate taken as a tablet – a brand name you may recognise is Clomid. It blocks oestrogen production, which in turn increases your production of follicle-stimulating hormone (FSH) by the pituitary gland to stimulate your follicles to grow mature eggs. You usually start taking the tablet on Day 2 to Day 6 of your menstrual cycle.

If the tablets don't work for you, then your doctor may prescribe injections of gonadotropin – follicle-stimulating hormone (FSH) and luteinising hormone (LH) – the hormones you need for ovulation.

You will be monitored (whether you are taking tablets or injections) by ultrasound scans to check the growth of the follicles, and blood tests to check the hormone levels in your blood. Once your follicles are an acceptable size you stop these injections and do an injection of human chorionic gonadotropin (hCG), commonly called the 'trigger shot,' which tells the follicles to release the mature eggs which is when ovulation occurs.

Depending on the reason why you are having this treatment, you will either be advised to have sex 12 to 36 hours after the trigger shot so sperm are waiting in the Fallopian tubes to hopefully fertilise an egg. If you have had OI in order to have IUI, this procedure will be scheduled for around 24-36 hours after the trigger shot. See 'Intrauterine Insemination' for more information.

Ovulation Predictor Kit (OPK)/Ovulation Predictor Test (OPT)

As the names suggest, these are kits or tests to help you to predict when you are ovulating. There are many different ones on the market so please do your research and read reviews as they aren't cheap and you may be using them for some time (though hopefully not).

Most work by detecting a surge in the luteinising hormone (LH) in your urine which occurs approximately 36 hours prior to ovulation (when you naturally develop and release an egg from one of your ovaries – see 'Ovulation' for more information). By having sex shortly after this surge for a couple of days, you increase your chances of getting pregnant.

There are pros and cons, as with anything, and some are listed here:

Pros

- if used correctly, they are pretty accurate at detecting the LH surge

- they are convenient as you use them on the days in the middle of your menstrual cycle

- they are easy to use – you pee on one of the test strips and the chemical on the strip gives you a result.

Cons

- they do not confirm that you have actually ovulated, they only tell you that you have had the LH surge

- they do not give you the date that you ovulated

- they don't take into consideration other factors involved in ovulation, such as your cervical mucus being of an egg white consistency

- they don't work if you have taken some fertility drugs

- they may not work reliably if you are over 40 because some women of this age have high levels of LH all the time

- they are of little use if you have irregular menstrual cycles or you have a hormonal imbalance such as PCOS.

You may want to use OPKs/OPTs as well as monitoring your basal body temperature (BBT) and observing your cervical mucus. Or you may want to use a monitor that measures your vaginal temperature, as this is the most accurate measurement of your core body temperature, so is very accurate in confirming ovulation and indicating your fertile window. See 'Ovulation' for more information.

Ovulatory Dysfunction

This is when you have irregular menstrual cycles and therefore ovulation is irregular, or you are not ovulating at all. Ovulation is when you naturally develop and release an egg from a follicle on one of your ovaries. If you have ovulatory dysfunction, your cycle usually ranges from 30 to 90 days or more. You may experience a milky breast discharge and have increased hair growth on your face and body.

Some of the causes are:

- excessive exercise

- obesity

- hormone issues such as hyperprolactinaemia, hypothyroidism, polycystic ovary/ovarian syndrome (PCOS), polycystic ovaries (PO)

- hypothalamic dysfunction, but this is less common.

The treatment will therefore depend on the cause:

- excessive exercise – ovulation can restart on its own by reducing the amount of exercise you are doing

- obesity – making nutrition and lifestyle changes can also bring about ovulation naturally without the need for medication

- hyperprolactinaemia, which is where you have high levels of the hormone prolactin which is produced by your pituitary gland – this may be due to a tumour which is usually benign and is treated with medication

- hypothyroidism, which is a disorder of your thyroid gland and is treated with thyroid replacement therapy – see 'Hypothyroidism' for more information

- PCOS, which is caused by excessive levels of male hormones – see 'Polycystic Ovary/Ovarian Syndrome' for more information

- Polycystic ovaries, i.e. when there is a higher number of follicles on your ovaries than normal – see this term for more information

- hypothalamic dysfunction, which can occur if you have a low percentage of body fat – treatment may be by taking progesterone or by diet/lifestyle changes.

A common treatment is to take the drug clomiphene citrate (Clomid) to encourage ovulation. For many this is the only treatment necessary, but if this doesn't work for you, there are other fertility drugs that might work. See 'Ovulation Induction' for more information.

Ovum/Ova

Ova is the plural word for 'eggs'. Ovum is one 'egg'. See 'Egg' for more information.

Ovum/Egg Donor Recipient

This means that you are using an egg or ovum donor to create your baby. You may need to use an egg donor because you cannot get pregnant using your own eggs despite having fertility treatment, or you may have had cancer treatment when you were younger, or have a genetic disorder that you do not want to pass onto your children. Alternatively, you may be a single man or a male couple who will need an egg donor to complete their family through surrogacy.

The egg donor will take drugs to stimulate her ovaries to produce more eggs than during a normal menstrual cycle, and these eggs will be collected and fertilised with either your partner's sperm, with your sperm or with a donor's sperm. See 'Egg Donor' for more information.

Oxidative Stress

For normal function and production, sperm produce small amounts of free oxygen radicals (ROS); this is normal for all the cells in our body. Their levels should be kept low so it is important that they are removed as soon as they have performed their function, and this is done by antioxidants. However, if there is an imbalance between ROS production and antioxidant activity, there will be high levels of ROS which cause oxidative stress. Unfortunately, sperm are very sensitive to oxidative stress, which can cause damage to the sperm cells and their DNA and lead to a decrease in sperm numbers and quality.

Causes of increased levels of ROS are:

- higher than normal levels of white blood cells in the reproductive system which can be a sign of infection or inflammation – pyospermia means semen that contains high levels of white blood cells

- increased scrotal temperature

- varioceles (varicose veins in the scrotum)

- cigarette smoke, alcohol and drug abuse.

To treat oxidative stress, if there is an infection it should be treated with a course of antibiotics. Also, lifestyle changes can be made regards smoking, alcohol and drugs, and a diet rich in antioxidants is also recommended.

As sperm are continually being made, once the oxidative stress has been reduced, the sperm numbers and quality should improve.

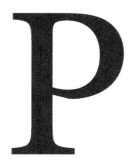

PELVIC INFLAMMATORY DISEASE

to

PROTOCOL

At age 30, your chance of a natural pregnancy is about 20% each month and your chance of pregnancy with in vitro fertilisation is about 42% each time you try.

Pelvic Inflammatory Disease - PID

This is an infection and inflammation of your pelvic organs including your womb, Fallopian tubes, ovaries and surrounding tissues. It is pretty common and is usually caused by a bacterial infection such as chlamydia and gonorrhoea that spreads from your vagina or cervix to your reproductive organs. It may not cause any signs or symptoms, or symptoms may be mild to severe.

Mild symptoms are:

- pain around the pelvis/lower abdominal area
- discomfort or pain during sex
- bleeding between periods and after sex
- a vaginal discharge that is yellow/green in colour.

More severe symptoms are:

- high temperature
- nausea and vomiting
- severe lower abdominal pain.

It is easily treated with antibiotics but if not treated, it can lead to scarring of your Fallopian tubes, which can cause infertility, ectopic pregnancy and pelvic abscess.

The below is not to scale and is an artistic impression of your reproductive system.

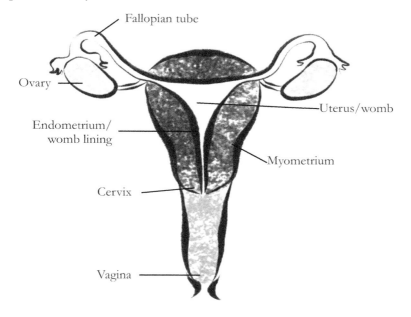

Percutaneous Epididymal Sperm Aspiration – PESA

In some men there is no sperm in their semen even though they ejaculate. The cause could be because the tube that carries the sperm from the testicle/testes is blocked, or it hasn't developed properly or sperm are not being produced at all. However, even if there is no sperm in their semen, there may be sperm or immature sperm in the epididymis (the tube sperm are stored in), or in his testicles.

PESA is a surgical sperm retrieval procedure where a fine needle attached to a syringe is inserted into the epididymis and fluid is sucked out. This would be the choice of retrieving sperm in men with obstructive azoospermia (no sperm due to an obstruction) as there is every chance that there will be sperm in the epididymis. It is a fairly quick procedure as there is no need to cut the scrotum or testicles.

If sperm are found they are then available to be used in fertility treatment, such as ICSI.

The below is not to scale and is an artistic impression of the male reproductive system.

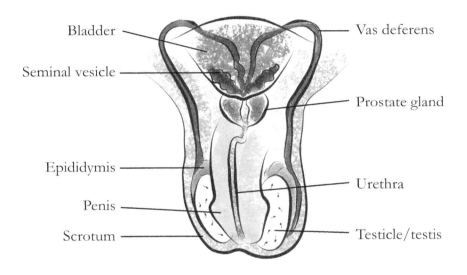

Perfluorooctanoic Acid – PFOA

This is a chemical that was used in the manufacturing of Teflon, which is the non-stick coating in cooking pans and other cookware. In addition, it can be found in microwave popcorn bags, upholstery, carpets and personal care products. It has the potential to be a health concern because it can stay in the environment and in our bodies for a long period of time. It is believed that PFOA can affect the time it takes you to fall pregnant.

Personalised Embryo Transfer – pET

This is the term used during ART such as IVF where an endometrial biopsy is performed in order to find out the exact day that your endometrium is at its most receptive to accept an embryo and for implantation to happen. See 'Endometrial Receptivity Array Test' for more information.

Pesticides

It has long been believed that pesticides interfere with our fertility, causing menstrual disorders, and men's infertility, resulting in lower sperm count and fewer normally developed sperm. Pesticides have also been blamed for causing miscarriages and premature birth.

Certain vegetables and fruit have a higher residue of pesticides than others, so the advice is to reduce eating so much of these – such as spinach, strawberries, peppers, grapes, kale, apples and tomatoes – or eat organic, and definitely always wash before eating. Alternatively, eat more fruit and vegetables that are lower in pesticide residue, such as avocado, beans, onion, plum, cauliflower and oranges.

Sheila says: There's something known as 'The Dirty Dozen' * regarding which fruit and vegetables have the highest levels of pesticides and which have the lowest, so if you want to know which are which, do a bit of research on the above term.

* Based on US Dept of Agriculture, so may vary in other countries.

Phthalates

These are a group of synthetic chemicals used to manufacture many everyday items such as plastic food containers, drinking bottles, cosmetics, fragrances, cleaning products and paints, to name a few. They are known as 'endocrine disrupters' which means they affect your hormones. The result of this means that it may take you longer to get pregnant and you may be more at risk of having a miscarriage and, if doing IVF or other fertility treatment, you may be more at risk of implantation failure.

Men's fertility may also be affected by phthalates in terms of sperm quality and reducing the levels of androgen hormones, particularly testosterone.

To avoid exposure:

- avoid cosmetics that have the ingredients DBP, DMP and DEP
- avoid plastic food containers or wrap that have a number 3 in the middle of the universal recycling symbol and the letters 'V' or 'PVC'
- do not store, heat or reheat food in plastic containers
- don't drink water from plastic bottles that have been left in the heat
- use natural body care products.

Pituitary Gland

This is a small, bean-shaped gland weighing less than one gram and is located at the base of the brain just below the hypothalamus. It is part of the endocrine system and produces follicle-stimulating hormone (FSH) and luteinising hormone (LH), both of which are concerned with your fertility and with a man's fertility.

In you, FSH acts on some of the follicles on your ovaries causing them to begin maturing at the beginning of your menstrual cycle. As the follicles continue to mature, the ovaries release increasing amounts of oestrogen/estrogen, which in turn tells the pituitary gland to stop producing FSH and instead release LH. The level of LH rises until there is a surge and the largest or dominant follicle releases its mature egg. This is ovulation.

Therefore, if the levels of these hormones are too low, as in a condition called hypopituitarism, your ovulation could well be affected. Treatment is by taking oestrogen/estrogen pills or wearing patches.

In men, LH acts on certain cells in the testes and stimulates the release of testosterone, the male sex hormone. FSH acts on different cells in the testes to stimulate the production of sperm. Therefore, if a man has hypopituitarism, his sperm production will be low or absent from a low amount of FSH, and a reduced amount of testosterone, causing:

- a lack of libido
- lack of energy
- loss of body/facial hair
- depression
- muscular weakness.

Treatment is by having testosterone injections.

Plastic

See 'Phthalates' for more information.

Polybrominated Disphenyl – PBDE

This was used as a flame retardant found in furniture cushions, fabrics, carpets, electronics and plastics. Although in many countries its use has been banned since the early 2000s, these household products may still be in use. If you or your male partner are exposed to high levels it can affect your fertility as some PBDEs mimic oestrogen/estrogen whilst others can block testosterone.

Polycystic Ovaries – PO

This is a condition you may be diagnosed with where your ovaries contain a large number – more than 15 – of harmless follicles that are up to 8 mm in size, as seen on an ultrasound scan. These follicles are referred to as 'cysts'.

It is not classed as a disease but may be a symptom of an underlying problem. It can be confused with polycystic ovary/ovarian syndrome or PCOS – see 'Polycystic Ovarian/Ovary Syndrome' for more information. It is more common in your late 20s.

It isn't completely clear what causes PO although the problems that cause PCOS also cause PO. Some experts think it is to do with having an underactive thyroid gland and that it leads to PCOS because of your eating and exercise habits. If you have PO, have no other hormonal issues and there are no male factor infertility issues, then you shouldn't have any problems starting a family.

Polycystic Ovaries Disease – POD
or Polycystic Ovary/Ovarian Syndrome – PCOS

This is a very common condition and it can affect you from as young as 15 years of age, and you are more at risk if you are obese or your mother, sister or aunt has PCOS. You may not have any symptoms and only find out you have PCOS when you are trying to get pregnant and are not succeeding. Common symptoms that you may get are:

- irregular menstrual cycles/periods of less than eight a year, more frequent than monthly or your periods stop completely
- an excessive number of follicles on one ovary or on both ovaries
- an excess of body hair (called hirsutism) on your face, chin and areas where men more commonly have hair
- acne or oily skin on your face, chest and upper back
- thinning hair or hair loss on your scalp
- weight gain or finding it hard to lose weight
- darkening and thickening of skin in your neck creases, groin and underneath your breasts.

The exact cause of PCOS is not known but it is thought to be genetic. The symptoms are caused by abnormal hormone levels, including high levels of insulin in your blood. Insulin is a hormone produced in your pancreas, which is located behind the lower part of your stomach and controls how the food you eat is changed into energy. If you have PCOS you may be resistant to the action of insulin, which means you do not respond normally to it. This results in your blood insulin levels being higher than normal. You are more at risk of developing insulin resistance if you have PCOS and you:

- are overweight or obese
- have an unhealthy diet
- do not do much physical exercise and
- have a family history of type 2 diabetes.

If the insulin resistance is not treated it can lead to you getting type 2 diabetes; the drug Metformin maybe prescribed.

Other health problems you are at risk of are high blood pressure, cholesterol could be affected, depression and anxiety and endometrial cancer.

Diagnosis is made by your doctor carrying out a physical examination, ultrasound scan and blood tests. If you have PCOS you can still get pregnant but it needs to be treated because the hormone imbalance means your eggs are not maturing and not being released from your ovaries, so you may not be ovulating.

There is no cure for PCOS, but you can manage the symptoms and help to regulate your periods by:

- making lifestyle changes – doing exercises, losing weight and eating healthily
- taking medication – to help you ovulate; a commonly prescribed drug is clomiphene citrate or Clomid – see Clomid for more information. If Clomid doesn't help you to become pregnant your doctor will probably suggest IVF – see 'In Vitro Fertilisation' for more information
- having surgery – a procedure called 'ovarian drilling' may help you to ovulate – see this term for more information.

Preimplantation Genetic Testing – PGT

This replaces two tests that were known as Preimplantation Genetic Screening, or PGS, and Preimplantation Genetic Diagnosis, or PGD. There are three categories: PGT-A, PGT-M and PGT-SR. See the following for more information.

Preimplantation Genetic Testing for Aneuploidy – PGT-A

This test specifically replaces Preimplantation Genetic Screening, PGS. A normal embryo has twenty-two pairs of chromosomes plus two sex chromosomes; forty-six in total. Aneuploidy is when there is an incorrect number of chromosomes in the embryo, for example forty-five or forty-seven, and these embryos are a cause of IVF failure and miscarriage. If an aneuploidy embryo does lead to a successful pregnancy, the baby is likely to have Down's Syndrome

Even if you do not have any fertility issues you will still need to do IVF, as once your eggs are collected and fertilised, the embryos can then be tested. See 'In Vitro Fertilisation' for more information. All twenty-three pairs of chromosomes are tested. Only an embryo with the correct number of chromosomes will be transferred into your womb. Any other embryos with the correct number will be frozen.

This type of test may be offered to you by your clinic if:

- you are over 35 years old

- if you have had previous miscarriages

- if you have had previous failed IVF cycles.

Preimplantation Genetic Testing for Monogenetic (single) Disease – PGT-M

This test specifically replaces Preimplantation Genetic Diagnosis, or PGD. PGT-M is a genetic test that has been designed to reduce the risk of having a child with an inherited disease. If you and/or your partner know you/they are a carrier, or you have a genetic disease that is due to a specific single gene or chromosome, such as cystic fibrosis, sickle cell anaemia, Duchenne Muscular Dystrophy or Huntingdon disease, during your genetic counselling you may be advised to have this test. Even if you do not have any fertility issues you will still need to do IVF, as once your eggs are collected and fertilised, the embryos can then be tested. See 'In Vitro Fertilisation' for more information.

Each PGT-M test is created specifically for the couple. After your eggs have been collected/retrieved and have fertilised, a small cell sample is removed by the embryologist from each embryo. This sample is then tested with your PGT-M test and an embryo that doesn't have the condition will be transferred to your womb. Any other unaffected embryos can be frozen.

Preimplantation Genetic Testing for chromosomal structure rearrangements – PGT-SR

This replaces the PGS translocation test. Translocation is when segments of two chromosomes (we all have 23 pairs of chromosomes; chromosomes carry our genetic information or genes), break off and change places. Therefore, this test identifies affected embryos. As with other PGT tests you will have to do IVF and cells will be removed from the embryos for testing. If you or your partner carry this translocation in your chromosomes, you may not know as you are probably healthy, but you may be having problems getting pregnant, have had failed implantations, a miscarriage or a baby who was stillborn, and/or have a child with a chromosomal abnormality which can lead to birth defects and intellectual problems.

Premature Menopause

The actual definition of menopause is your last period. Premature menopause is when your menstrual periods stop before you are 45 years old. Some countries may give the age as 40 but either way, it's before the natural age you would expect to get the menopause, which is around 50 years old. The main cause is that your ovaries stop producing eggs and stop making normal levels of hormones, mainly oestrogen/estrogen. Other causes include:

- chromosome abnormalities
- if you have an autoimmune disease
- if you have had chemotherapy or radiation
- if you have had your ovaries removed
- if there is a family history of early menopause.

Other terms that are more often used by fertility experts when you are trying to get pregnant are 'premature ovarian ageing', 'premature ovarian failure' and 'primary ovarian insufficiency' – all explained under 'Premature/Primary Ovarian Insufficiency' in this book. Unfortunately, there doesn't seem to be one agreed international term.

Premature Ovarian Ageing – POA

See 'Premature/Primary Ovarian Insufficiency' (below) for more information.

Premature Ovarian Failure – POF

See 'Premature/Primary Ovarian Insufficiency' (below) for more information.

Premature/Primary Ovarian Insufficiency – POI

This is a decline in the function of your ovaries before you are 40 years old; in some cases, it can be as early as adolescence. This loss of ovarian function and therefore reduced fertility is due to a premature reduction in the number of ovarian follicles or follicles not responding to follicle-stimulating hormone (FSH) and luteinising hormone (LH), often for unknown reasons. Because the functionality of the ovaries is not efficient, not enough oestrogen/estrogen is produced so your pituitary gland reacts by trying to make more FSH to try and stimulate the ovaries to produce more oestrogen/estrogen. However, your ovaries often don't stop working completely and you may still occasionally have a period and ovulate, so you can get pregnant years after being diagnosed.

Having POI means that you are more at risk of reduced bone density leading to osteoporosis (thinning of the bones) because of the reduction in oestrogen, and also cardiovascular conditions. You are also more at risk of developing hypothyroidism, namely Hashimoto thyroiditis, and also a high chance of getting adrenal insufficiency.

There are a number of reasons for POI and in a majority of cases there is no known cause, which can be devastating news to hear, and is especially difficult knowing you may not be able to have children at all or that you will probably require fertility treatment. Counselling should be offered as it is known that a diagnosis of POI is highly likely to cause emotional distress and affect self-esteem.

The known causes are:

- autoimmune disorders – your body's immune system attacks your tissues and organs, such as your ovaries

- genetic causes – especially abnormalities in your sex female chromosome, or X chromosome, or other genes that affect the sex hormone functionality

- following pelvic surgery or a hysterectomy

- following chemotherapy and radiotherapy for cancer

- environmental toxins such as pesticide, pollutants, smoke and chemicals.

The symptoms are the same as if you were starting the menopause. Along with irregular menstrual periods or no periods, you also may experience:

- hot flushes/flashes

- night sweats

- vaginal dryness

- irritability

- trouble sleeping

- low sex drive

- unexplained infertility.

A diagnosis is made following your doctor taking your medical history of irregular (for at least three months) or no menstrual periods. They will also send you for an ultrasound scan to determine the number of follicles and the size of your ovaries and ask you to have some blood tests – if you are having periods they will need to be done at the beginning of your menstrual cycle but if you aren't, they can be done on any day of your cycle. You will also have these tests done twice, at least four weeks apart. The blood tests are:

- follicle-stimulating hormone (FSH) – this will be higher than normal (over 30iu/l)

- oestrogen/estrogen level will be very low

- luteinising hormone (LH) will be higher than expected but not as high as FSH

- testosterone level will be lower than normal

- thyroid function test to check levels and

- anti-Müllerian Hormone (AMH) levels are usually lower than normal. See 'anti-Müllerian Hormone' for more information.

There is a small chance that you will get pregnant naturally, especially if you are still having periods, even though they may be irregular. You may be happy to wait and see if you can get pregnant naturally. However, if you are not having periods at all or want to start a family, you may need to consider IVF. You may be able to do IVF initially with your own eggs and see if it is successful, or your doctor may suggest you use donor eggs.

Most countries have online support for POI either from a charity or a Facebook group, and these are very good places to seek help if you're struggling with accepting your diagnosis.

Primary Infertility – PI

The World Health Organisation (WHO) defines this as when a woman has never been able to get pregnant or has never carried a pregnancy and delivered a live baby.

The WHO also states that infertility in women is ranked the fifth highest serious global disability (among populations under the age of 60).

See 'Infertility' for more information.

Progesterone – Prog

If you are not producing the correct amount of the hormone progesterone, it will be very difficult or impossible for you to get pregnant.

Progesterone is produced as the follicles that contain the immature eggs start to develop on the ovaries. Progesterone levels rise in the second half of your menstrual cycle and when the mature egg pops out of your ovary (i.e. ovulation), the ovarian tissue that replaces the follicle, known as the 'corpus luteum', continues to produce progesterone as well as oestrogen/estrogen. Its main function is to thicken your womb lining (endometrium) in order to enable a fertilised egg to implant, and then to nourish the embryo and establish the placenta – which will take over producing progesterone until your baby is born.

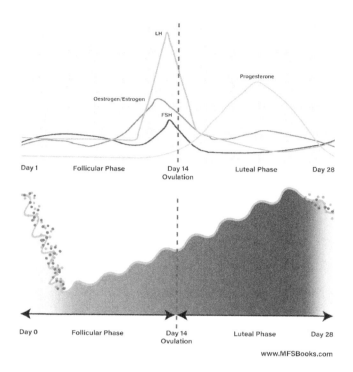

www.MFSBooks.com

In some of us we don't make enough or we make too much progesterone. This has a number of implications:

- ovulation doesn't happen
- a fertilised egg doesn't implant
- your endometrium cannot support your pregnancy.

A number of things can cause irregular progesterone levels, such as too much oestrogen/estrogen, pollution, eating meat and their by-products from animals that have been fed hormones, or eating too much soy (or other foods that contain natural plant oestrogen, or phytoestrogens). See 'Xenohormones' for more information.

If you have too much progesterone, you may experience the following:

- anxiety

- trouble concentrating
- irregular periods
- low libido
- fatigue and tiredness
- sore breasts
- weight gain
- headaches
- insomnia.

If on the other hand you produce too little progesterone to maintain a pregnancy, you may experience the following:

- scanty or absent menstrual cycles
- recurring early miscarriages
- vaginal dryness
- hot flushes/flashes
- depression
- foggy memory
- endometriosis
- swollen breasts.

There are a couple of relatively easy ways to find out if your levels of progesterone are correct:

1. Record your basal body temperature daily as this will show if your temperature spikes around the time you ovulate. If you don't get a spike, it could be a sign that you are not producing the correct amount of progesterone. See 'Basal Body Temperature Charting' for more information.

2. If you ovulate less than 11 days before your menstrual

period starts, this could be a sign that you are not producing enough progesterone which will affect your womb lining from thickening.

3. Your doctor may do a blood test to check your progesterone levels, if they don't, ask for one.

4. Another method is to do a saliva test first thing in the morning - this is when the daily hormone production has peaked.

If your results show a progesterone imbalance, there are some things you can do to correct this imbalance and once your body is producing the correct levels (providing there is nothing else that is affecting you or your partner's fertility), you stand a better chance of getting pregnant. Some suggestions are:

1. You can reduce your exposure to xenohormones (oestrogen/estrogen-mimicking compounds) found in solvents, adhesives, plastic, meat, dairy, pesticides and soap, to name a few.

2. Apply progesterone cream to your skin – the best areas are neck, upper chest, breasts, palms of hands and soles of feet. It is absorbed by your skin into the underlying fat and then into your bloodstream. Please seek medical advice – do not self-medicate.

3. Take the herb Chasteberry - it is believed to help balance progesterone and oestrogen/estrogen imbalances. Before taking any herbs etc you must seek expert advice – do not self-medicate.

If you are doing ART such as IVF, donor egg IVF or frozen embryo transfer (FET), you will be prescribed progesterone in some format. This is because when doing something that is unnatural, as the above is, your body needs lots of progesterone to prepare your womb lining for the transferred embryo/blastocyst to implant, and to stay the whole nine months. Post-IVF etc, you will be prescribed progesterone as a pill, vaginal suppository, injection into the muscle, or a smaller needle injection into the fat just under the skin (subcutaneous) – which one you are prescribed is down to your clinic's preference but be sure to talk to your team if you have strong feelings about one type or another.

Progesterone in Oil – PIO

This is a daily progesterone injection into your muscle, usually your buttocks or thigh, that you may be prescribed following IVF, ICSI, donor egg IVF or frozen embryo transfer (FET). The injection can be painful and it is not uncommon to get a rash from the oil. See 'Progesterone' (above) for more information.

Prolactin

This is a hormone with over 300 functions in your body; it regulates your immune system, metabolism and reproductive system to name a few. It is mainly produced in the pituitary gland in your brain but also in your uterus and breasts. Prolactin production is controlled by two hormones: dopamine and oestrogen/estrogen. Oestrogen/estrogen tells the pituitary gland to begin production of prolactin whilst dopamine tells it to stop production of prolactin.

If you have too much prolactin (hyperprolactinaemia), this can cause problems with your fertility. See 'Hyperprolactinaemia' for more information.

Protocol

This is the plan of treatment that you follow with your doctor's advice when you are doing fertility treatment, such as IVF. You may follow a 'long protocol' or a 'short protocol', and the main difference is the length of time from when you start your treatment up to the stimulation of your ovaries. Long protocol is approximately four weeks whereas the length of time for the short protocol varies, but is less than four weeks. See 'In Vitro Fertilisation' for more information.

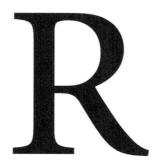

RADIATION
to
RUBELLA

A typical adult uterus/womb weighs about 60 grams.

Radiation

This treatment uses high-energy rays to kill cancer cells and these rays can damage your reproductive organs. If you are having radiation therapy to your abdominal or pelvic region, then some of the radiation will be absorbed by your ovaries and could destroy some or all of your eggs, or bring on the menopause early. Damage to your ovaries can be prevented by having minor surgery to move your ovaries out of the targeted treatment area. Your ovaries absorb a high dose of radiation if the targeted area is your vagina.

If you are having radiation to your womb, this can cause scaring which will reduce the blood flow to your womb. This can result in a higher risk of miscarriage, a low-birth weight baby and a premature baby, especially if you had radiation therapy as a child before your womb had properly developed.

Your pituitary gland may be affected if you are having radiation therapy to your brain and, as the pituitary gland is involved in ovulation (when an egg is released from your ovary), this may affect your fertility.

If your partner is having radiation therapy, depending on where the targeted area is, he may also be at risk of infertility. If the therapy is directed at his testicles, his abdominal area or in his pelvic region, it could kill the stem cells that produce sperm.

The hypothalamus and pituitary gland may be affected if he is having radiation treatment to his brain. They are responsible for producing luteinising hormone (LH) and follicle-stimulating hormone (FSH) which tell the testicles to make testosterone and sperm – therefore his sperm count could be affected.

The UK charity Cancer.org states: 'Studies have suggested that women with cancer are less likely to be given information about preserving their fertility than men.' This means you may need to bring up the subject with your doctor in case they don't mention it.

Rainbow Baby

A baby born alive and well following a previous miscarriage or stillbirth. It denotes the rainbow after a storm.

Reciprocal IVF

You may also see this referred to as 'partner IVF' and it is an option for a lesbian couple where both can play a part in the conception of their baby/babies – one produces the egg/eggs and the other carries the baby. If you are producing the eggs, you will go through an IVF cycle. Once your eggs are collected/retrieved, they will be fertilised with the donor sperm you have both selected. At the same time as your ovaries are being stimulated, your partner's menstrual cycle will be aligned with yours so that her womb lining is ready for the embryo to be transferred into her. Then you both wait for two weeks to find out if it's successful.

The main difference with reciprocal IVF and IVF between a heterosexual couple or single woman is that between you, you need to decide which of you will provide the eggs and who will the embryo be transferred into. This may be a simple decision, such as:

- if one of you is much younger, then your eggs have a better chance of the IVF being successful

- general health and fitness

- desire to experience pregnancy and giving birth may be stronger in one of you.

All the emotions and ups and downs are exactly the same, regardless as to who does IVF – whether you are a lesbian couple, a gay couple, single, or a heterosexual couple. Everyone wants to get pregnant and have their longed-for baby and everyone should be supported and listened to in exactly the same way. Nowadays, there are many different places to get support that is more geared towards your particular circumstances – this could be someone blogging, running a Facebook group or a support group run by a fertility clinic or fertility expert.

Depending on the country that you are doing the IVF in, this is the same as donor egg IVF so there may be legal requirements.

Recurrent Implantation Failure – RIF

You may receive slightly different figures as to what 'recurrent' means as it varies in different countries. The European Society of Human Reproduction and Embryology (ESHRE) defines it as: 'Failure to achieve a pregnancy after three completed fresh IVF-ET cycles.'

Causes of RIF are either down to your embryo or to your endometrium (womb) lining, such as:

- poor egg/sperm quality
- poor embryo quality
- chromosomal abnormalities in the parents
- your womb lining not being ready to receive an embryo
- adhesions in your womb
- immunological factors
- thrombophilia or blood clotting issues.

If you experience RIF it is distressing and devastating and you will understandably turn to your clinic for answers. Your clinic should offer you counselling and you should not be rushed into making decisions straight away about future treatment, but you may wish to discuss such things as:

- lifestyle changes, such as giving up smoking (if you and/or your partner smoke) and/or alcohol and losing weight

- preimplantation genetic testing or next generation sequencing for chromosomal abnormalities

- assisted hatching

- changing to short IVF protocol or to long IVF protocol

- endometrial receptivity array or ERA

- sperm DNA testing

- endometrial scratch.

All the above terms are explained fully in this book.

You may decide to change clinics and you are within your rights to do this. Even if you have frozen embryos at the clinic, these can be transferred to another clinic of your choice.

Sheila says: When we did our second ICSI cycle in Spain and I miscarried, I went into research overdrive about RIF. We decided to have some further tests done and our clinic in Spain agreed to support us in this decision and with the medication I was then on. So, it does often help to be open and honest with your clinic but also to take ownership of your journey. Had our clinic not agreed, we had no hesitation in going elsewhere. We will always be grateful to them for being supportive and working with us.

Recurrent Pregnancy Loss – RPL

This is defined as the loss of two (in some countries like the US), three (in the UK), or more consecutive pregnancies. Going through one miscarriage is distressing but having one miscarriage after another is devastating and soul destroying. You will probably dread the thought of trying again and it feels like an uphill struggle, especially when many around you are seemingly getting pregnant without any problems. Even when you do get pregnant, you don't want to get too excited or tell anyone because you are afraid you may miscarry again.

It is advisable that you have investigations into what could be causing you to miscarry every pregnancy as it is possible that, if you have treatment, you will go on to have a successful pregnancy and deliver your baby. Some causes of recurrent miscarriage are:

- abnormal chromosomes in one of you or both of you; you should both have a blood test where this can be tested for and if the results show a problem, you will be referred to a specialist

- hormonal imbalance that causes other conditions, such as polycystic ovaries – see 'Polycystic Ovaries' for more information

- problems with your uterus, such as if it is abnormally shaped – this would be found out during an ultrasound scan

- if you have a blood clotting disorder, such as systemic lupus erythematosus or SLE, or anti-phospholipid syndrome. Although these conditions are rare, if you are suffering from one of them it will cause your blood to clot and could be affecting the normal functioning of the placenta. This would be found out by you having a blood test and treatment is blood-thinning medication. See 'Anti-phospholipid Syndrome' for more information.

This is it extremely important that you have support during this awful time, both you and your partner (if applicable). Trying to get pregnant when it is challenging takes over your life, and to cope with miscarriage after miscarriage is undoubtedly going to affect you and those around you. It is a fact not many people know that you can suffer from post-traumatic stress disorder (PTSD) after a miscarriage. Most countries will have a charity for supporting you if you have had a miscarriage and they are usually run by people who have also had a miscarriage, so it is very often worth contacting them.

Reflexology

This dates from the ancient Chinese and Egyptians and works on the principle that you have 'reflexes' on your feet that are linked to organs and systems within your body, such as your Fallopian tubes and ovaries. A reflexologist massages these different points on the soles of your feet to unblock the energy pathways to help your body to regain its natural balance. In doing so, you experience a deep relaxation which may help to reduce stress and calm your mind.

Reflexology may help to:

- balance your hormones
- regulate your menstrual periods
- help with ovulation
- improve blood circulation.

It may also help increase sperm quality and quantity by counteracting the negative effects of stress.

As with acupuncture, there are no real studies that have been undertaken, so whether reflexology will help you or not is inconclusive. Please be sure to seek the advice of an expert in this area and if you are wanting to do reflexology, or any other holistic treatment during fertility treatment, please let everyone involved know.

Reproductive Endocrinologist – RE

This is an obstetrician/gynaecologist (OB/GYN) who has then specialised in those endocrine disorders specifically concerned with infertility in men and women. You may be referred to a RE after seeing your own doctor and they will carry out fertility tests and investigations in order to diagnose and treat you appropriately.

Reproductive Immunologist

An immunologist is a scientist or physician who has studied further and now specialises in the immune system, specifically diagnosis and management of diseases, such as autoimmune diseases and allergies. A reproductive immunologist will focus on how your immune system and your reproductive system interact, both when you are trying to get pregnant and when you are pregnant. You may be referred to one if you have unexplained infertility, have had recurrent miscarriages or if you have had unexplained recurrent IVF failures.

Reproductive Surgeon

They will have previously trained as a gynaecologist or a urologist and specialises in female or male reproductive surgery. You would be treated by one if you needed surgery to remove fibroids or to treat endometriosis for example.

RESOLVE

This is the non-profit National Infertility Association in the US that was established in 1975. It supports and empowers, by knowledge, those people who are finding it challenging to build their family. It works to raise awareness of infertility, works with the US government on fertility issues, offers advice to US citizens about paying for fertility treatments and so much more.

Rubella

Also known as 'German measles', this is more often thought of as a childhood illness, but adults can get it too. In some countries like the UK, it is very uncommon because children are immunised against it, but this may not be the case in other countries.

Before you start fertility treatment you will have to either have a blood test to check your immunity or show your clinic a copy of a previous test result. The reason for this is that if you get pregnant and you then catch rubella in the first twenty weeks of pregnancy, you could have a miscarriage or your unborn baby could be stillborn, or have birth defects, such as deafness, brain damage, heart defects and cataracts.

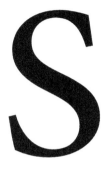

SAUNA/STEAM ROOM

to

SURROGATE/SURROGACY

Around 15% of all adult males, up to 35% of men who are evaluated for male infertility and around 80% of men who are infertile due to some other cause have varicoceles.

(figures from 2012 & 2015)

Sauna/Steam Room

This is relevant to the men because sperm don't like it hot. There is a reason why a man's testicles are on the outside of his body, and it's so that the sperm being produced inside don't get overheated. It is understood that using a sauna/steam room lowers sperm count and reduces motility (the ability to swim in a straight line). Fortunately, both count and motility will improve (providing there is no other cause) if the man doesn't use a sauna or steam room for at least three months; which is the length of time it takes to make new sperm.

Scar Tissue

Also called 'adhesions' and 'synechiae', these are bands of fibrous tissue that may form in your womb, on your ovaries or your Fallopian tubes. They are caused by:

- previous gynaecologic pelvic surgery; even surgery to remove scar tissue
- by infections such as chlamydia and gonorrhoea
- by diseases, such as endometriosis and pelvic inflammatory disease, or PID.

It is likely to be harder for you to get pregnant if you have scar tissue in your womb because the blood supply to your womb lining, or endometrium, will be decreased, so you won't have a healthy endometrium, which is what an embryo needs in order to implant. See 'Asherman's Syndrome' for more information.

Diagnosis is by hysteroscopy or laparoscopy – see both these terms for more information. Scar tissue can be removed surgically and this can increase the likelihood of you getting pregnant, but the surgical procedure needs to be carried out with care in order to prevent more scar tissue from forming following the surgery.

Secondary Infertility – SI

This is when you are unable to get pregnant or to carry your baby to term after previously having had a child, or children, after a year of unprotected sex if you are younger than 35, or after six months if you are 35 or older. It is almost as common as primary infertility (when you've not been able to get pregnant after at least one year of having unprotected sex), and is very confusing and bewildering, especially if you fell pregnant very quickly the previous time(s).

The causes are similar to primary infertility:

- male infertility, such as low or no sperm count, problems with sperm shape or movement, blockage in the tubes that carry the sperm during ejaculation, issues with the hormones or glands involved in sperm production
- ovulation problems whether irregular or absent
- damage to your Fallopian tubes
- problems with your womb, such as fibroids, or your womb lining
- endometriosis
- complications following your previous pregnancy/ies or delivery/ies
- recurrent miscarriages
- lifestyle changes since your last baby was born, such as weight gain, smoking and medications
- you (and your partner) are older
- other, unexplained causes.

Often you put off going to see your doctor for many reasons: you keep trying, as you've had one or more children and you think your doctor won't be interested in helping you; others tell you not to waste the doctor's time as you have your family; and so on. The truth is, regardless whether you are trying for number two or number five, you have the same feelings about it being a struggle to get pregnant as someone who doesn't have any children – anxiety, stress, jealousy, pain, grief, to name a few.

The tests and investigations you need will be the same as those for primary infertility (all of these are explained in this book):

- blood tests for hormone levels for you both

- semen analysis for your partner (if you are not using a sperm donor)

- hysterosalpingography

- possibly a sperm DNA test

- possibly an ovarian reserve test.

Treatment will depend on the outcome of the test results but you may:

- need to make lifestyle changes

- take hormone medication to help you ovulate

- have surgery to assist with your fertility.

If you are using your partner's sperm, he may need surgical sperm retrieval and you may need IUI, IVF or donor egg or sperm. Again, all these treatments are explained in this book.

If you do need fertility treatment, how you feel emotionally and about yourself is again the same as someone who has never had a baby, and if you don't find the support you need from family and friends there are threads on fertility forums for secondary infertility, there are Facebook groups and often fertility clinics have a support group specifically for people experiencing secondary fertility.

Semen Analysis – SA

Also called a 'sperm count' or 'seminogram', this is the first test carried out on the man when investigating infertility, as it evaluates various characteristics of his semen and the sperm in the semen.

It goes without saying that he is going to be very anxious about doing the test and getting the results, just as you are. He'll see it as a reflection on his manhood just as some women feel guilt that their body is letting them down when they can't get pregnant.

The sample can be collected either in a private room at your doctor's/clinic, where it will be sent off directly to the laboratory, or he can collect the sample at home in a container provided by the doctor. If doing it at home the sample must be delivered to the laboratory within one hour. No lubricant should be used as this could affect the sperms' ability to move. He must also tell the doctor if he is taking any medication or health supplements. He will be advised to not have sex or to masturbate two to seven days before providing the sample.

The sample will be looked at under a microscope in the laboratory and the results will cover the areas detailed below. The figures stated are from the World Health Organisation (WHO) in their 2010 guidelines. You may find your fertility clinic has different amounts that they consider are normal, and unfortunately it is common, where fertility is concerned, to not have everyone agreeing on test results.

Semen volume – the lowest level that is considered 'normal' is 1.5ml. As 96-98% of semen is water, one way of increasing the volume is to drink more fluids.

Total sperm number – this is the total number of sperm in the sample and a normal number is 39 million per ejaculate.

Sperm count/concentration – this is measured in millions of

sperm per millilitre of semen – a normal count is over 15 million/ml.

Motility – this is how the sperm are moving and at least 50% should be active 60 minutes after the ejaculate was produced. Some reports may grade the sperm as follows:

- 'a' or 'IV' have progressive motility and are the strongest and fastest swimmers

- 'b' or 'III' are classed as 'non-linear motility' and travel in a crooked movement

- 'c' or 'II' are non-progressive, which means they are not moving forwards despite moving their tail

- 'd' or 'I' are immotile and aren't moving at all.

Morphology – this is the size, shape and appearance of the sperm and 4% or more of the sperm must be normal – anything less would indicate a problem with the sperm fertilising your egg. Abnormal sperm can be a result of genetic issues, infection, exposure to toxic chemicals and an increase in the temperature of the testicles.

Colour of the semen – this is assessed because if it isn't a whitish-grey colour it could indicate infection, inflammation or that he could have a sexually transmitted disease.

pH of the semen – this is important because if it is too acidic (low pH), or too alkaline (high pH) it is harmful to the sperm. The normal range is 7.2-7.8.

Liquefaction time or viscosity - this measures how long it takes for the semen to change from thick and sticky (which is what it is like at first and sticks to your cervix), to more liquid or watery which enables the sperm to swim better. The expected time is 15-20 minutes but providing it is within 60 minutes, this is normal. If it doesn't change this could affect the sperms' ability to swim to your egg.

Vitality/viability - this refers to the percentage of live sperm in the ejaculate and a normal percentage is at least 58% are live sperm.

If the results come back and indicate there are fertility issues, it is really important to tell the doctor about anything that could have affected the sample, such as recent illness, a visit to the sauna, medications or stress over doing the test. He will probably be asked to do the test again in approximately four weeks' time. As sperm are constantly being produced, making lifestyle changes may positively affect future test results. See 'Sperm' for more information.

Sheila says: Sometimes it really helps to have a laugh at funny things that happen when everything around you seems horrible. When my husband did his very first semen test, we decided that he should do it at home. We kept putting it off, as you do, until one day we decided today was the day. I looked at the test request form the doctor had given him and there were only certain days the hospital accepted samples, and today was the last day until the next week. Plus, it had to be received at the lab within one hour from the time it was now! You can only imagine what went on in our house next and what the drive to the hospital was like! Everything is pretty grim where sperm samples are concerned sadly, from the room the guy has to go into at the clinic, to how he feels and to the letterbox for 'samples' – at our hospital it certainly made you think 'shifty men in raincoats'! We laughed about this for ages after.

The below is not to scale and is an artistic impression of a sperm.

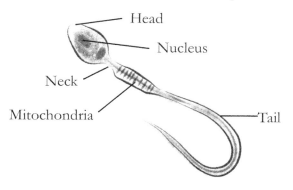

Head

Nucleus

Neck

Mitochondria

Tail

Semen/Seminal Fluid

This is the fluid that a man ejaculates during sex or when masturbating and we probably assume that it is only made up of sperm swimming in a sticky fluid. However, this isn't quite correct. It is made up of secretions from three sets of glands;

1. The prostate gland produces about 30-35% of the total seminal fluid; because it is alkaline, this neutralises the acids that naturally exist in the urethra and vagina which prevent the sperm being killed off

2. The seminal vesicles (two glands that sit above the prostate) make about 65-70% of the total seminal fluid; this is also alkaline and contains fructose (a type of sugar), which gives the sperm energy to swim up your womb to the Fallopian tubes. It also contains citric acid, free amino acids, enzymes, potassium, zinc, prostaglandin and phosphorylcholine

3. Cowper's glands (two pea-shaped glands just beneath the prostate) together with fluid from the testes make about 2-5% of the total seminal fluid.

The seminal fluid analysis is as important as the other factors that are tested in a semen analysis because it can help to identify what specifically is causing infertility, such as blockages and problems with specific parts of the male reproductive tract, as well as infections. All should be treatable with surgery, medication or fertility treatment such IUI. See 'Semen Analysis' for more information.

Semen pH

The normal pH of semen is alkaline at 7.2-8.0. A higher or lower pH can indicate problems in the prostate gland and seminal vesicles, and could very likely be harmful to sperm and affect their ability to fertilise your egg.

Seminologist

The person at the clinic who only deals with semen and sperm and is responsible for semen analysis, freezing and storing of sperm for fertility treatments.

Septate Uterus

Also called 'arcuate' uterus, this is a congenital abnormality in the shape of your uterus. Your uterus should be the shape of an upside-down pear: big at the top and skinny and tapered where it meets your cervix. This should also be its shape inside if an egg is going to implant and successfully grow into your baby. In a septate uterus, a thin membrane divides your uterus either partially or fully from top to bottom. As this involves the top of your uterus, known as the fundus, this may make implantation more difficult because this is the area where the fertilised egg prefers to implant.

More commonly it will cause you to miscarry, and often it's every pregnancy and more usually when you are over 12 weeks pregnant. You may well not realise that you have a septate uterus until you have investigations into recurrent miscarriages, and then it may be diagnosed when you have an ultrasound or a hysterosalpingogram and/or hysteroscopy.

It is treated with surgery usually during a hysteroscopy and can be done as an outpatient. It is fairly minor but is delicate because the amount of membrane that needs removing is tiny and scarring of your uterine lining is a risk. However, if you do have the surgery your chances of carrying a baby to term are very much increased.

Serum Progesterone Test

This is a blood test to measure the amount of the hormone progesterone in your blood. See the term 'Progesterone' for more information.

Sex Hormone Binding Globulin – SHBG

This is a protein that is made mostly by your liver, with smaller amounts being made in your brain, womb and placenta when you are pregnant, and in men in their testes/testicles. SHBG binds itself to the sex hormones testosterone and dihydrotestosterone (DHT) in men and oestradiol (an oestrogen/estrogen) in you, and carries them in your blood in an inactive form. Its role is to carry these three hormones to other tissues in your body and it plays an important part in maintaining the balance between oestrogen/

estrogen and testosterone in your body. Optimal SHBG levels decrease your risk of developing PCOS, insulin resistance and type 2 diabetes.

The level of SHBG can be tested by doing a blood test, and in men it is used to check for testosterone deficiency which means the SHBG level would be raised. For you, the test is a helpful tool to find out if you have high levels of testosterone, which means you would have low levels of SHBG, which in turn could indicate that you have PCOS.

The best way to improve your low levels of SHBG is to treat your PCOS-related insulin resistance and improve the PCOS hormones. See 'PCOS' for more information.

Short Protocol Cycle

This is the term used by your fertility clinic when you are starting an IVF cycle, and the 'short' part refers to the length of time that you are taking medication for before your eggs are collected/ retrieved. You may be advised to follow the short protocol if:

- you have had OHSS in a previous cycle

- your ovaries haven't responded well in previous cycles and you did the long protocol

- you are older, so in your late 30s.

Your treatment usually starts on Day 3 of your cycle when you have an ultrasound scan and/or blood test to check that the lining of your womb has thinned out. Providing that it has, you start doing the injections that will stimulate your ovaries to produce lots of eggs, known as 'stimulation'. You will have regular scans until your follicles and womb lining show that you are ready for egg collection/retrieval.

At this point you will follow the same path as a long protocol and do the 'trigger' hCG injection (human chorionic gonadotropin) approximately 36 hours before egg collection/retrieval.

The advantages are that you take fewer drugs, it doesn't take as long from start to end, it is cheaper as fewer drugs are involved and you may produce more eggs (though this is not always the case). See 'In Vitro Fertilisation' for more information about the whole process.

Single Embryo Transfer – SET

See 'Elective Single Embryo Transfer – eSET' for more information.

Sleep

The quality and quantity of sleep you get every night may be affecting your fertility because disrupted sleep patterns cause hormonal imbalance, low basal body temperature (BBT) and suppress ovulation. Sleep affects your key fertility hormones, namely oestrogen, progesterone, luteinising hormone (LH) and follicle-stimulating hormone (FSH). Regular sleep is necessary to produce proper amounts of the hormone leptin and, as leptin affects ovulation, disrupted sleep may cause irregular menstrual cycles.

If you work night shifts it is a known fact that you are likely to have disrupted menstrual cycles because your internal clock, known as the 'circadian rhythm', is confused and doesn't know whether it's day or night. This internal clock is controlled by regular patterns of light and dark within a 24- hour period, but this is no longer regular when you do night shifts as you sleep during the day and have days off when you sleep at night. This affects the production of the sleep hormone melatonin and the stress hormone cortisol. The key is to try and bring about hormonal balance and regular menstrual cycles by:

- making your bedroom completely dark when you sleep during the day

- getting out into the daylight without any sunscreen/block for at least 15-20 minutes when you are working nights so you get some Vitamin D.

If you generally find it hard to sleep at night or have difficulty falling asleep, you may want to think about:

- meditating before sleep

- keeping a journal/diary to see if there is something that you do during the day/evening that could be affecting your sleep

- not having food or drink too near bedtime

- not using a mobile phone/laptop/tablet or watching TV too near the time you go to bed.

Smoking

You are probably very aware that smoking when you are pregnant can affect your unborn baby. But it is also now known that smoking and/or passive smoking can also affect your fertility. You are more likely to take longer to get pregnant than a non-smoker and each stage of conceiving is affected:

- it can damage the DNA of your eggs

- it can affect the ability of your eggs to mature which may affect ovulation

- it can disrupt production of your reproductive hormones

- it can alter how receptive your womb is to enable a fertilised egg to embed.

You are also more at risk of having a miscarriage when you do get pregnant or of having an ectopic pregnancy. You may also be affecting the fertility of your unborn child.

Where men are concerned, smoking can also affect their fertility in the following ways:

- it can cause erectile dysfunction

- it can damage the DNA in his sperm due to 'oxidative stress', which can affect the health of your unborn child

- it can prevent his sperm from maturing

- the volume of seminal fluid is less

- sperm production will be lower because he has a lower concentration of proteins in his testes/testicles that are needed for producing sperm, so his sperm count is lower

- the percentage of sperm with good motility (ability of sperm to swim forwards in a straight line) is lower.

If you are considering starting fertility treatment, especially something like IVF, most clinics will refuse to treat you if one or both of you are still smoking. This is because smoking could reduce the number of eggs you produce, increase the possibility of fewer eggs fertilising and affect an embryo successfully implanting. The advice is to stop smoking at least three months before trying to get pregnant but at least one year is even better and much safer for any baby/babies that are born.

Social Egg Freezing

This is when you freeze your eggs for reasons that are not to do with an illness, disease or treatment that could damage your fertility in the future. Egg freezing has been around since the early 1990s for preserving the fertility of young women having cancer treatment. Social egg freezing is aimed at women in their 20s and 30s who, for a number of reasons, are not ready to have a baby now but would like to have their own biological baby sometime in the future. Because your eggs age as you do, the younger the eggs are, in theory, the better chance you have of getting pregnant when you want to.

In order to freeze your eggs, you have to have your ovaries stimulated to produce more eggs than the one egg that is normally produced during your natural menstrual cycle. This means you have to go through the first stage of an IVF cycle and inject hormones, and you may have to do more than one cycle to get a good quantity of eggs. There is a risk that your ovaries could overstimulate and you get OHSS, which can be life threatening. Once your eggs have been collected they are frozen or 'vitrified'. Some countries have a restriction on the length of time eggs can be frozen for; in the UK it is ten years but longer in special circumstances.

Sometime in the future when you want to get pregnant, some of your eggs will be thawed and hopefully they will fertilise and develop into embryos and a baby. But there is no way of knowing, at the time of freezing, what condition your eggs will be in when they thaw. If an egg is fertilised, you will have the embryo or blastocyst (a five-day old embryo) transferred back into your womb, and hopefully it will implant and develop normally, so you have your baby nine months later.

This is a very 'hot' topic, with some people being very much against freezing eggs for social reasons and others being very much in favour.

Society for Assisted Reproductive Technology – SART

This is an organisation of professionals who are dedicated to the practice of assisted reproductive technologies or ART, such as IVF, in the United States of America. Their mission is to set up and help maintain standards of ART. More than 90% of fertility clinics in the US are members of SART and these clinics meet the highest standards for safety, quality and patient care.

Society for Reproductive Endocrinology and Infertility – SREI

This is an affiliated society of the American Society for Reproductive Medicine, or ASRM. Reproductive endocrinologists are obstetrician-gynaecologists who have an advanced education, and research and professional skills, in reproductive endocrinology and infertility. They treat reproductive disorders and male and female infertility. The members of SREI are dedicated to providing excellence in reproductive health through research, education and care of patients.

Sonohysterogram

Also called a hysterosonography, sonohysterography or saline sonohysterogram, this is an ultrasound of the inside of your uterus. It is one of the first investigations you may have done as it will show the doctor if you have any abnormalities in your uterus that may be stopping you from getting pregnant.

It takes about 15 minutes and can be done at your clinic, at your doctor's or in hospital. You may want to take a couple of painkillers before you have it done as it can cause cramping during the procedure. It is best carried out a week after your period ends as this is when your endometrial lining (the lining of your uterus) is thin and the risk of infection is minimal.

It is similar to having a pap/smear done as a speculum is inserted into your vagina so that the doctor can see your cervix. A thin plastic catheter is then passed through your cervix into your uterus, the speculum is removed and the transvaginal ultrasound or 'wand' is slowly inserted into your vagina. A small amount (about 10ml) of sterile saline (salt and water solution) is slowly passed through the catheter into your uterus, which makes it easier for the doctor to see, via the ultrasound, inside your uterus and to view the lining. Once it is finished, the 'wand' and catheter are removed. Some of the saline solution will be absorbed and some of it will come out of your vagina.

Sonosalpingography

See 'Sononhysterogram' (above) for how the procedure is carried out.

The difference between a sonohysterogram and sonosalpingography is that during the ultrasound the Fallopian tubes are investigated to see if they are unblocked, as the saline solution will be seen to flow along the tubes.

Spanish Fertility Society

This is a scientific society in Spain that aims to promote studies on fertility and to support its application to social problems that are related to it. One objective is to advise the administration and other relevant groups on issues relating to reproductive health as well as passing on appropriate knowledge.

Sperm

Also called a spermatozoon (plural spermatozoa), this comes from the Greek word 'sperma' meaning 'seed'.

When a baby boy is developing in your womb, specialised cells called 'germ cells' move to the gonads which are in the testes/ testicles. During puberty, the cells begin to divide, producing sperm. A sperm is the smallest cell in a man, being 0.05 mm from head to tail, and has three parts:

1. A head that contains enzymes – to break through the egg membrane – and the DNA and chromosomes

2. A midpiece which is where the sperm's energy (mitochondria) is stored

3. A tail which moves the sperm forward to travel through your cervix and womb to your Fallopian tubes in order to fertilise an egg.

Each sperm contains 22 chromosomes plus either an X or a Y chromosome making 23 in total, which is the same as an egg. Therefore, it is the sperm that determines the sex of the baby – a sperm with an X chromosome will create a baby girl, and with a Y chromosome will create a baby boy.

The fluid that carries sperm is called 'semen' so, although we think it's sperm that is ejaculated, it's actually sperm in semen. The semen/sperm travels from the testicles, through tubes called vasa deferentia and out through the urethra during an ejaculation.

Over a man's lifetime, he will produce billions of sperm and they can live up to five days after ejaculation in your Fallopian tubes. Although only one is needed to fertilise an egg, the WHO (World Health Organisation) guidelines in 2010 stated that a normal sperm count is fifteen million or more per ejaculate, anything less may cause problems in conceiving.

If sperm are damaged this can cause fertility problems and sperm are at risk of being damaged in the following ways:

- oxidative damage from laptops, mobile phones and toxins in the environment
- by very hot environments, such as sauna/steam room, heated car seats, laptops
- a man's lifestyle – if he smokes cigarettes, drinks more than the recommended amount of alcohol, drinks a large quantity of coffee (caffeinated), has a diet poor in nutrition and is overweight.

Luckily men are continually making sperm and as it takes about 70 days for a sperm to fully mature, it means that if a man makes lifestyle changes, he can produce better quality sperm a few months later, providing there are no other issues that are causing the sperm to be damaged.

The below is not to scale and is an artistic impression of a sperm.

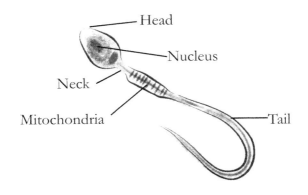

Sperm Agglutination

This is to do with the percentage of sperm stuck or clumped together in a sperm sample. When sperm are stuck together they cannot swim very well, and they need to be able to swim in order to reach and fertilise an egg.

In a test result, the percentage of sperm agglutination refers to the percentage of sperm that are stuck together in the sample. The most common cause of sperm agglutination is following an infection or due to anti-sperm antibodies because the antibodies stick together. During ART, sperm would be washed so they are no longer clumped together. See 'Sperm Washing' for more information.

Sperm Analysis – SA

See 'Semen Analysis' for more information.

Sperm Bank

This is a facility or a company, sometimes in a fertility clinic or in a hospital, which properly collects and stores sperm from sperm donors. In the UK, they are governed by the Human Fertilisation and Embryology Authority (HFEA), which has rules and regulations about the collection, storage and use of sperm donations in order to protect the donor and the recipient, and to ensure that any babies that are born from the sperm are healthy. In the USA they are regulated as Human Cell and Tissue or Cell and Tissue Bank Products (HCT/Ps) establishments by the Food and Drug Administration (FDA). Many states have additional regulations over and above those from the FDA. In Europe, they must have a licence according to the EU Tissue Directive.

It is really important that you ask at the sperm bank you contact in your country, or the country where you are getting your sperm from, that they are registered, and about their rules and regulations. You should ask:

- how they do their background checks on donors
- if they complete a full medical history and whether they go back at least one generation
- how they collect and store the sperm
- if the donation is anonymous or not – some banks will only do one type whilst others will do both. See 'Sperm Donor' for more information.

Sperm banks are used for a number of reasons, such as:

- where the man has a problem with his sperm which means you won't be able to get pregnant with his sperm
- in unexplained infertility
- if the man has a genetic condition that he doesn't want to pass onto any children he fathers
- by a single woman who wants to conceive a child of her own
- by a lesbian couple who want to conceive a child of their own.

Some sperm banks will only deliver sperm to a doctor/clinic whereas others will deliver to your home.

Sperm Count

According to the World Health Organisation (WHO) guidelines

in 2010, fifteen million sperm per ml (or higher) of semen is considered a normal count.

Sperm DNA Testing

Inside each sperm is the DNA from the man. From the moment the sperm are made in his testicles to the time it takes to fertilise an egg – quite a long period and a vast distance to travel – the DNA can become damaged or fragmented.

The traditional semen or sperm test doesn't look at the internal structure of the sperm, which is where the DNA is located, and even a normal semen analysis test could contain sperm with DNA fragmentation. Often if a couple have 'unexplained infertility' or recurrent miscarriages it is due to sperm DNA fragmentation. It is believed that the fragmentation can occur due to oxidative stress – see 'Oxidative Stress' for more information.

By carrying out an additional DNA fragmentation test alongside the semen analysis, it is easier for your doctor to advise the correct treatment if there is a higher level of fragmentation diagnosed. Initially this may be some lifestyle changes, such as giving up smoking, taking an antioxidant supplement, so that newly produced sperm have less DNA fragmentation.

Sperm Donor – SD

This is a man who donates his sperm with the intention that it will be used to enable you to have a baby. You may be single, may have a partner who has problems with his sperm or you may be in a lesbian relationship. A sperm donor may be known to you or they may be from a sperm bank you select to use.

If a man is donating through a sperm bank he may not have a say in who uses his sperm. A man who donates mostly does it for altruistic reasons and not for monetary gain. It doesn't pay as much as egg donation and he usually only receives payment for expenses and, in some cases, for inconvenience.

In some countries is it the rule that a sperm donor receives counselling prior to donating so that he knows exactly what is involved and, if applicable, that he may be contacted in the future by children born as a result of his donation. You as the recipient should also fully discuss what is involved, and what problems could arise in the future. Not everyone is comfortable with bringing up a child that they are not biologically related to. This may be even more important if you are using a known donor.

If you are considering using a sperm donor it is extremely advisable that you contact a sperm bank rather than just searching online or via an advert. This is because reputable sperm banks are regulated. Even if you do know the donor, he should still have tests – see below. See 'Sperm Bank' for more information.

A sperm donor is generally between 18 and 35 or 45 in some countries. A background check is completed by the sperm bank to ensure his medical and family history is correct. He will be screened for infectious diseases, such as:

- HIV-1 and HIV-2
- syphilis
- chlamydia
- gonorrhoea
- hepatitis A and B virus
- cytomegalovirus

and hereditary diseases, such as:

- cystic fibrosis

- sickle cell anaemia

- thalassaemia

- congenital adrenal hyperplasia.

His sperm will also be tested to ensure that it is healthy and will be good for donating. An initial sample will be frozen and then thawed to check that the sperm survive the thawing process. The sperm bank usually guarantees the quality and amount of motile sperm in a thawed sample. If he is then accepted as a sperm donor by the sperm bank, his sperm will be constantly monitored, he will be regularly checked for infectious diseases and his blood will be tested regularly. He must agree to give up all legal rights to any children that result from his donations. He must also produce future sperm donations at the bank so the bank knows that he is producing the sperm and not another man. It also means that his donation can be processed immediately. His donation is stored in small vials or straws of between 0.4-1.0ml of sperm and is cryogenically preserved (or frozen) in liquid nitrogen tanks.

The sperm bank will create a profile for each sperm donor and these are either online for you to look through or are only available if you are having treatment with them. This means that you can learn a little bit about them, as well as check their medical history. In some countries, the information you will know about the donor is quite limited, such as skin colour, ethnicity, eye colour, height, weight and blood group. At some sperm banks you may be able to pay for additional information about the donor, such as age, education and family history. In the UK most donors are anonymous and you will only know the same information as detailed above. However, any child that is born as a result of the donation can, when they reach 18 years old, request the donor's name, date of birth and last known address from the HFEA. This will be different for all countries.

Once you have selected a potential donor, his semen will be tested to ensure that you and he are a good match.

The donor isn't told your identity but if they want to know if any children have been born, they may be told depending on the country's regulations. The sperm bank's own rules limit the number of pregnancies a donor can achieve and this is the reason a donor is only allowed to make no more than a certain number of donations. In the UK, (this may be different for other countries), a donor is not allowed to create more than ten families, where the number of children in that family can be any number. Realistically, most donors create one or two families of one or two children.

Sperm Freezing

This will preserve a man's fertility, either for his own use in the future or for someone else to use to create their family, as in sperm donation. A man may decide to freeze his sperm if:

- he has a medical condition or is about to start treatment that may affect his fertility

- the quality of his sperm is deteriorating

- he has difficulty producing a sample on the day of the fertility treatment, such as IUI or IVF.

If a man is going to freeze his sperm, he must sign a written consent and decide how long he wants the sperm frozen for. Once he produces his sample, it is mixed with a special fluid to protect the sperm from any damage during freezing and is divided between a number of vials or straws, so in effect there are a number of treatments available if need be.

Treatment with frozen sperm is just as successful as treatment with fresh sperm and there are no risks to future children. In the UK the storage period is normally 10 years though it can be for up to

55 years in certain circumstances.

Sperm is then flash-frozen using a process called 'vitrification' as the motility and survival of the sperm is much better than the previous slow freezing method.

Sperm Morphology

See 'Semen Analysis' for more information.

Sperm Motility

See 'Semen Analysis' for more information.

Sperm Test

You may see 'sperm test' mentioned on forums etc and you may see 'sperm tests' for sale – this is the general word used for the male fertility test that checks his semen and the sperm in the semen. The correct name for the test your clinic or doctor arranges is a 'semen analysis' – see this term for a full explanation of what is involved in this test.

Sperm Washing

This is a common process in fertility clinics prior to fertility treatments such as IVF and IUI. Once the sperm sample has been produced, it is 'washed' in the laboratory, meaning that chemicals, mucus and non-motile sperm are removed from the semen, and sperm are separated from the seminal fluid. Doing this procedure improves the ability of the sperm to fertilise the eggs.

The below is not to scale and is purely an artistic impression of the procedure 'sperm washing' (of course it isn't like this at all!).

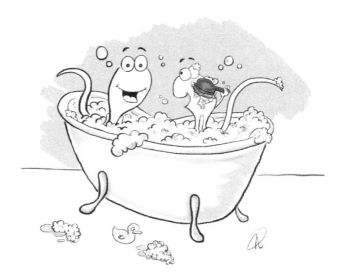

Steroids

These drugs, whether prescribed or taken as body-builders (anabolic steroids), can affect your fertility and a man's fertility. If you take steroids, it can cause irregular menstrual periods which will then affect ovulation. For men, the result of taking anabolic steroids could be erectile dysfunction and lowered sperm count. This is because steroids cause the testicles/testes to shrink, which means that sperm are no longer being produced. If high doses are used for a long time, the damage can be permanent.

Stimulation – Stim

This is referring to your ovaries being stimulated during fertility treatment, to mature more than the one follicle and egg that matures during your natural menstrual cycle. Within your ovaries are hundreds of thousands of follicles and each one contains an immature egg. During your natural menstrual period several of these follicles begin to develop as a result of the release, from the pituitary gland in your brain, of a hormone called follicle-stimulating hormone or FSH. One of these follicles will become a dominant one which grows faster than the others, and it is the egg in this dominant follicle that is released during natural ovulation.

The drugs used for ovarian stimulation vary depending on the type of fertility treatment you are having and your clinic's preference.

Some side effects of ovarian stimulation are:

- nausea
- feeling bloated
- hot flushes/flashes
- headaches
- mood swings
- a condition called OHSS – see 'Ovarian Hyperstimulation Syndrome' for more information.

When you are going through this part of fertility treatment, you will be carefully monitored by ultrasound scan and blood tests so that your doctor can vary the dosage of your medication, observe how many follicles are growing and how your womb lining is thickening.

This part of fertility treatment is always nerve wracking because you live for every scan and are on edge to find out how many follicles are growing. If you are on forums where others are at the same stage of treatment as you are, it is very hard not to compare how you are doing to how they are doing. It's hard but try and remember that quality rather than quantity is more important. For more information – see 'In Vitro Fertilisation'.

Stress

Very few people would argue that finding it challenging to have a baby and/or doing fertility treatments isn't stressful. After all, life is carrying on around you as if nothing is different and you still have to go to work (which may also be stressful), pay the bills which are higher if you are paying for your fertility treatment, and see your family and friends announcing that they are pregnant (so stressful). What the experts can't agree on is if stress itself causes fertility issues; though many do agree that it does cause anxiety and depression.

Your body is equipped to deal with everyday stresses that come and go – it's known as the 'fight or flight' response, and if you experience an actual or perceived harmful event, attack or threat, your adrenal glands (located right above your kidneys) make extra adrenaline – a stress hormone. This has the result of quickening your heart rate which increases the amount of blood pumping round your body to your limbs but away from your reproductive organs, so you can literally fight or run for the hills. Then, when the actual or perceived harm has gone, your adrenaline levels return to normal.

Research has shown that when stress hormone (such as adrenaline and cortisol) levels are high, this can stop the release of your body's gonadotropin-releasing hormone (GnRH), which in turn is responsible for the production of your sex hormones. The results may be any of the following:

- irregular menstrual cycles

- poor follicle production

- lack of ovulation due to increased levels of cortisol and prolactin

- progesterone production is affected which is needed for implantation to happen

- levels of follicle-stimulating hormone (FSH) rise

- interest in having sex decreases in you and in men

- low sperm count.

If you think you may be stressed, it's quite likely that you are and it isn't the best way to live your life, whether you're doing fertility treatment or not. If you can, think about some 'me' time and consider some of the following therapies that help to reduce stress – and most are actually quite pleasant:

- acupuncture

- meditation

- reflexology - find someone experienced in fertility reflexology

- fertility yoga

- emotional freedom technique or EFT

- counselling and

- neurolinguistic programming (NLP).

Subcutaneous injection – S/C

Some fertility drugs are taken as injections. This type of injection gives small amounts of medication into the fat layer between your skin and muscle. The needles are smaller than intramuscular injections. You can do a s/c injection into the following parts of your body:

- abdomen, about 5cms on either side of your belly button
- thigh, between your knee and hip and slightly to the side.

It's a good idea not to give the injection in exactly the same spot each time as you may get some slight bruising and skin irritation.

Super Ovulation

This is another term for 'ovarian stimulation'. See 'Stimulation' for more information.

Support Group

It is now understood that women and men going through fertility investigations and treatment can really benefit from support that is available in a number of different ways, be it an online forum, a Facebook group or a face-to-face group. A support group:

- is a place you can share how you feel
- is a place where you can hear from other people who understand what you are going through, which reassures you that you are not alone
- offers understanding because the people in the group have been through or are going through fertility struggles
- offers practical information to support you.

A number of clinics have set up face-to-face support groups for people having treatment at their own clinic and also for people having treatment elsewhere. Also, some women or couples themselves have set up groups that meet at the pub for example, and other fertility experts, such as coaches, acupuncturists and nutritionists have also set up face-to-face groups for local women and men.

Most people don't want to talk about the fact that they are having problems getting pregnant as it is very personal and a lot of times they don't want to worry their families and friends. Those nearest and dearest to us aren't always the best for providing the support we so desperately need – despite well-meaning intentions.

As there are nowadays a number of different ways to get support, you really can choose the one that suits you best because, as with everything to do with fertility, no one size fits all.

Surgical Sperm Retrieval – SSR

In some men, when a semen analysis is performed, the results show that there are no sperm in the ejaculate or a very small number. The reasons for this could be:

- sperm are being made in the testes/testicles but there is a block in the vas deferens (one of the two tubes that carry the sperm) as a result of infection or injury

- there is no van deferens due to a congenital abnormality

- the man has had a vasectomy

- non-obstructive azoospermia.

If this is the case, sperm can hopefully be collected directly from the testes using various surgical techniques, such as 'Percutaneous Epididymal Sperm Aspiration' (PESA), or 'Testicular Sperm Extraction' (TESE). See either of these for more information.

Any sperm that are retrieved by either of these methods are frozen. If it is necessary for your partner to have PESA or TESE it will be carried out before your egg collection. This is just in case no sperm are retrieved. If sperm are collected and frozen, they will be thawed and ready when your eggs are collected and the probable fertility treatment you will have will be ICSI rather than IVF.

Surrogate/Surrogacy – Surr

This is when a woman carries and gives birth to a baby for someone else: a heterosexual or lesbian couple, a single woman or man or male same-sex couples. Where it is because the woman has a medical condition or it is impossible or dangerous for her to get pregnant and give birth, the reasons may be:

- womb abnormality or no womb
- cardiac issues
- recurrent pregnancy loss
- recurrent IVF failure.

There are two types of surrogacy:

1. Partial, straight or traditional – this is when a surrogate's egg is fertilised with sperm from the intended father. This is usually done using artificial insemination, either at home or at a clinic. See 'Traditional Surrogacy' for more information.

2. Full, host or gestational – this is when eggs from the intended mother or a donor are used, so this will have to be done using IVF. See 'Gestational Surrogacy/Carrier' for more information.

Some people who need to use a surrogate may ask a family member or a friend, and this can work very well as you all obviously know each other. If, however you need to look further, there are agencies in many countries who allow surrogacy, and each country will have their own laws and regulations. If you do travel abroad and your surrogate has a baby, getting a passport and the baby back into the UK, for example, can be a difficult and time-consuming process. In most countries you will need to apply for a parental order when you return with your baby to the country that you live in. This is because the surrogate is recognised as the legal parent.

It goes without saying that neither the intended parent/s nor the surrogate go into surrogacy without giving it a lot of thought first as there is so much to consider. Everyone involved should receive counselling before, during and after the birth, and be open and honest about their expectations and what they don't want to happen. However, if done correctly and sensibly, it can give everyone involved a lot of pleasure and a future they only dreamed of.

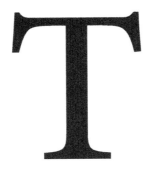

TESTICLES/TESTES

to

TWO-WEEK WAIT

The highest pregnancy rates occur if sexual intercourse occurs the day prior to ovulation, with rates declining if intercourse occurs on the day of ovulation.

Testicles/Testes

These are the male reproductive glands that are in the scrotum, which is the sack that hangs down just behind the penis. They are oval shaped and their job is to make and store sperm and to produce the male sex hormone testosterone. One testicle (or testis) is usually bigger than the other and is it not uncommon for one to hang slightly lower than the other. They are usually up to 2 inches long, 1.2 inches in height and 0.8 inches across. Inside each testicle are very fine coiled tubes called 'seminiferous tubules' and it is here that the sperm start to develop from puberty.

The temperature of the testes is very important because if it is too high or too low, this affects sperm production, so it is maintained at 35°C (95°F), which is two degrees below normal body temperature. The smooth tissue of the scrotum moves the testicles closer or further away from the body if necessary.

It is at about six weeks of pregnancy that the baby's sex organs either develop into those for a girl, i.e. ovaries, or those for a boy, i.e. testicles. The testicles start to develop in the baby's abdomen and by the time the baby is born, they have usually moved down to hang outside the body in the scrotum. Sometimes only one descends by birth and the second has usually descended within three to six months of age. Sometimes neither descend and this is known as 'undescended testicles' – see this term for more information.

The below is not to scale and is an artistic impression of the male reproductive system.

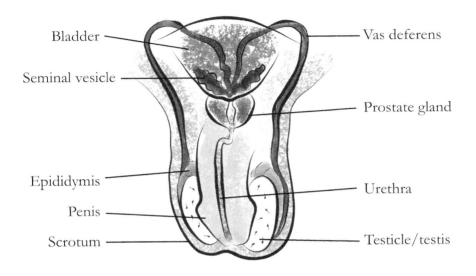

Bladder

Seminal vesicle

Vas deferens

Prostate gland

Epididymis

Penis

Scrotum

Urethra

Testicle/testis

Testicular Biopsy

See 'Testicular Sperm Extraction' for more information.

Testicular Sperm Aspiration – TESA

This is a procedure where sperm is retrieved (aspirated or sucked) directly from the testicles/testes and is commonly used if a man has 'obstructive azoospermia', where a blockage is the cause of sperm being absent from his semen.

It is usually carried out under a local anaesthetic using a fine needle for the aspiration. There is usually some swelling and pain following the procedure.

Testicular Sperm Extraction – TESE

When a man has no sperm in his semen but the vas deferens (small tube that carries the sperm) is not blocked, this usually means there is a problem with sperm production and he will be diagnosed with 'non-obstructive azoospermia'. This could be due to:

- a genetic condition that affects his fertility
- having had chemotherapy or radiotherapy
- having had a testicle removed
- surgery as a baby to bring down an undescended testicle.

It is unlikely that there is a large number of sperm so aspirating, as in the case of TESA (above), would not be the correct procedure. Instead, an incision is made into the testicle to remove a small portion of tissue from the testicle and any viable sperm are then extracted from this tissue. Where multiple samples of tissue are taken from different areas of the testicles, this is called 'multi-site TESE' and is done under general anaesthesia.

An alternative procedure called 'micro-TESE' maybe performed instead and it is also carried out under general anaesthesia but involves examining the testicles with a microscope to find areas or tubules where sperm are being produced. These tubules are removed and, if possible, the sperm extracted. Rest and painkillers are advised for a couple of days after the procedure.

Testosterone

This is the main male sex hormone and it:

- plays a role in the development of male reproductive tissues, such as the testes/testicles

- is key for normal sperm production

- is responsible for bringing about secondary sexual characteristics, such as growth of body/pubic hair and a deep voice

- ensures that muscle and bones stay strong during and after puberty

- enhances his sex drive

- is also concerned with health and well-being.

It is mainly produced by the testicles/testes with a smaller amount being produced by the adrenal glands (they sit on top of the kidneys).

Luteinising hormone (LH), which is produced in the pituitary gland in the brain, tells the testes to produce testosterone, which travels around the bloodstream doing all the things mentioned above. The brain monitors the blood levels of testosterone and if they get too low (known as hypogonadism), the brain stimulates more LH to be produced. The opposite happens when testosterone levels are too high, if for example, performance enhancing drugs are taken: the brain reduces or stops the production of LH.

Testosterone levels are naturally at their highest in the morning and gradually reduce as the day goes on.

When investigating infertility, a blood test may be carried out to measure the levels.

Although it is the main sex hormone in men, it is also produced in much smaller quantities by your ovaries and adrenal glands and is important for:

- bone strength

- development of lean muscle mass and strength

- overall sense of well-being and energy

- your sex drive.

If you have high levels of testosterone, you may have:

- excess facial hair

- acne

- some balding

- irregular menstrual cycles

- mood changes

- be overweight.

Raised levels in you are commonly due to PCOS. See that term for more information.

Three-Person IVF

This is the term commonly used, often by the press, for 'mitochondrial donation treatment' or 'mitochondrial replacement'. Every cell, including your eggs, has mitochondria which are responsible for converting the energy from the oxygen we breathe in and the food we eat into the energy that powers our cells. In order for the cells to function correctly, the mitochondrial genes need to be working properly or the cells can die, and brain, heart, lung and muscle function can be severely affected, causing life-threatening diseases that worsen with age. Although men's cells also have mitochondria, it is mitochondria gene abnormalities in your eggs that could be passed onto any children you have.

In 2016 a baby boy was born with 'genetic information from three people' in Mexico and in January 2017, a baby girl was born with DNA from three people in the Ukraine where this technique was used for the first time.

In 2015 in the UK mitochondrial donation was made legal and is regulated by the Human Fertilisation and Embryology Authority (HFEA). Currently there are two techniques – 'maternal spindle transfer' (MST) and 'pronuclear transfer' (PNT):

1. Maternal spindle transfer – your genetic material, i.e. your genes that make you who you are, is removed from your eggs that are collected/retrieved following IVF and transferred into donated eggs (hence 'three-person'), which have had their genetic material removed. The eggs are then fertilised with sperm in the fertility clinic's laboratory and will hopefully develop into embryos.

2. Pronuclear transfer – your eggs are collected/retrieved following IVF and are fertilised with sperm in the fertility clinic's laboratory and hopefully will develop into embryos. The genetic material from each embryo is then transferred into embryos that have been created by donated eggs from a third person and sperm from your partner, or from a donor. The genetic material will have been removed from the donated eggs.

The embryos that are transferred back into your womb will contain your and your partner's (or sperm donor's) genes, which means that the child that is born will be your biological child but will not have the abnormal mitochondria because it has been replaced with the donor's healthy mitochondria. Both techniques work equally well.

In the UK if you know that there is a high chance of you passing on a serious mitochondrial disease to your children, then mitochondrial donation may be an option for you. You will have to be assessed by the fertility clinic(s) that are licensed in the UK by the HFEA as only people who are at a very high risk of passing on a serious disease to their children are eligible for this treatment. If your clinic thinks that you are eligible they then apply to the HFEA for permission to go ahead with the treatment, because the HFEA has to approve every case to ensure it is only carried out in a legal and ethical way. If you want to find out more because you think you might be eligible, you can contact one of the UK's three main mitochondrial disease centres in London, Oxford or Newcastle.

Because it is such a new technique, if you do have mitochondrial donation treatment, your clinic will ask if they can follow up on your child's health and development as this will help doctors to understand, as much as possible, the effects on children born following this treatment and on future generations. You don't have to agree but if you do you will be helping many people in the future affected by mitochondrial disease.

A cautionary note: this technique might not be 100% efficient as it is believed that even when this technique is used, a tiny number of abnormal mitochondria can still be transferred to the embryo.

The below is not to scale and is an artistic impression of an egg.

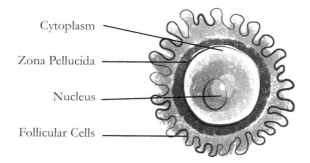

Cytoplasm

Zona Pellucida

Nucleus

Follicular Cells

Thrombophilia

This is a condition where your blood clots and can obstruct the blood flow to vital organs such as your heart, brain and lungs. It can be inherited or caused by:

• surgery

- obesity

- pregnancy

- taking birth control pills

- long periods without moving, such as on a flight

- a condition called 'anti-phospholipid syndrome' or APS. See 'Anti-phospholipid Syndrome' for more information.

Often you don't know you have thrombophilia but it you have a family history of clotting disorders such as strokes, deep vein thrombosis (DVT) or blood clots in the lungs, you may be more at risk and can have blood tests carried out to determine this. Also, if you have PCOS you may be more at risk of blood clots because of the high insulin resistance.

Some fertility experts believe that if you have thrombophilia this may cause you to have miscarriages and implantation failure following fertility treatment. These experts would prescribe blood-thinning medication to prevent further miscarriages and implantation failures.

Thyroid Gland

This is a butterfly-shaped gland that partially surrounds your windpipe and is part of your endocrine (hormonal) system, which is under the control of your hypothalamus and pituitary gland in your brain. The main hormones produced by your thyroid gland are thyroxine (T4) and small amounts of triiodothyronine (T3). Thyroid-stimulating hormone or TSH stimulates the thyroid gland to produce these two hormones.

Every cell in your body is dependent on thyroid hormones for:

- regulating metabolism – the chemical process that occurs in our cells so that we continue to live

- managing blood calcium levels

- producing energy

- metabolising fat

- using oxygen

- maintaining your weight

- balancing other hormones.

The health of your thyroid can be affected by:

- being exposed to environmental toxins, such as pesticides, chemicals, heavy metals such as fluoride and mercury, and electromagnetic radiation

- high stress levels

- autoimmune disorders

- infections

- inherited conditions from your parents

- nutrient deficiencies, especially too much or too little iodine

- hormonal imbalances, such as oestrogen and prolactin.

An underactive thyroid, known as 'hypothyroidism', or an overactive thyroid, 'hyperthyroidism', could be the reason you are struggling to get pregnant, and especially so if you have been given a diagnosis of 'unexplained infertility'. Treating the thyroid gland may mean that you can get pregnant naturally, if there are no other fertility problems. You (and your partner) should have your thyroid levels tested as part of your fertility tests.

If you have poor thyroid health, where your fertility is concerned, you may experience the following:

- irregular or absent menstrual cycles

- ovulation is absent (even though you are having menstrual

periods) due to thyroid hormone levels not being ideal, and so affecting the level of luteinising hormone (LH) which is needed for ovulation to occur

- short luteal phase due to low levels of LH which lowers the production of progesterone which is needed to thicken your womb lining (endometrium), resulting in a fertilised egg not implanting

- lower basal body temperature (BBT) due to low thyroid function, meaning that the temperature range for the implanted embryo is not correct, so its cells cannot rapidly divide so may be unable to grow, which could result in an early miscarriage

- too high levels of thyrotropin-releasing hormone (TRH) and low levels of thyroxine (T4) resulting in excess production of prolactin which effects your fertility by preventing ovulation, or causing you to have irregular or absent menstrual periods

- mood changes and tiredness, which can affect your libido.

Men's fertility is also affected by hypothyroidism or hyperthyroidism in the following ways:

- lowers sperm production

- affects sperm motility (ability to move) and morphology (appearance)

- sperm DNA damage due to oxidative stress

- reduced testosterone levels

- reduced sex drive

- erectile dysfunction.

The thyroid tests you should have carried out if you are having problems getting pregnant and have symptoms of hypo or hyperthyroidism are: TSH, total T4, free T4, total T3 and free T3.

It is important to get any thyroid issues sorted prior to getting pregnant because you are more at risk of miscarriage and, when your baby is developing in your womb, s/he is at risk of:

- low birth weight

- being born prematurely

- impaired growth and development of the testicles in a baby boy.

Correcting hypothyroidism is usually by taking a thyroxine medication but you should also look at eating foods that are good for thyroid health, namely colourful vegetables and fruit, healthy proteins, fats and wholegrains and food rich in iodine, such as seafood, eggs and strawberries. If you are interested in the holistic approach, you may want to seek expert advice on herbs that support your thyroid and adrenal glands. It is very important that you don't self-medicate and you always seek the advice of your healthcare professional.

Thyroid-Stimulating Hormone – TSH

The hypothalamus and the pituitary gland, which are in your brain, regulate thyroid function by communicating with each other to ensure the balance of the two main thyroid hormones – thyroxine (T4) and triiodothyronine (T3) – is maintained.

The hypothalamus produces thyrotropin-releasing hormone (TRH), which tells the pituitary to produce more or less TSH. TSH directly tells the thyroid gland to produce correct amounts of T3 and T4 depending on the levels of these two hormones in your bloodstream. If your T3 and T4 levels drop, your pituitary gland produces and releases more TSH, which tells your thyroid gland to produce and release more T3 and T4. If, however, your T3 and T4 levels are too high, your pituitary gland releases less TSH, which tells your thyroid gland to slow down producing T3 and T4.

If your thyroid is producing too much T3 and T4 so you have low levels of TSH, you have a condition called 'hyperthyroidism', and if your thyroid gland is not producing normal levels of T3 and T4 so you have high levels of TSH, you have a condition called 'hypothyroidism'. See 'Hyperthyroidism' and 'Hypothyroidism' for more information.

When all these hormones that are associated with your thyroid gland are unbalanced, other hormones that are essential for your fertility are affected, such as follicle-stimulating hormone (FSH) and luteinising hormone (LH), which could mean it will take you longer to get pregnant or, if your levels are not checked, it could mean that you are misdiagnosed.

Your TSH level, which is actually checking your pituitary gland and not your thyroid gland, should ideally be between 0.4 and 2 mIU/L (again, this may vary depending on the country you live in).

Thyroxine – T4

This is the inactive hormone your thyroid gland releases into your blood. It travels to organs such as the liver and kidneys where it is converted into its active form of triiodothyronine or T3. T4 (and T3) affects the function of practically every organ and cell in your body, such as your:

- heart
- digestion
- metabolism – the chemical process that occurs in our cells so that we continue to live
- brain development

- bone health

- muscle control

- general health and well-being.

If you think you have thyroid disorders, you should have a blood test for T4 and T3 levels. See 'Thyroid Gland' for more information.

Time-lapse Monitoring

Also called 'embryo monitoring' and there are various brand names that you may read on websites/forums etc. What they do is the same: they monitor and record – sometimes as often as every five minutes – the embryo's development in the laboratory.

It is believed by some experts that, by recording the embryos as they develop, the embryologist is able to make a more informed decision as to which embryos have developed normally and which will be the best to transfer into your womb. By monitoring with one of these time-lapse pieces of equipment, the embryos are not removed from the incubator so they do not experience any change in temperature or humidity.

You will come across experts who believe time-lapse embryo monitoring is a great step forwards and those who believe that it makes no difference as to it helping to select the best embryo for transfer. Not all clinics offer it so, if it is something you are really keen on, remember to ask your clinic.

The below is not to scale and is purely an artistic impression of embryo development.

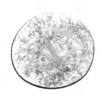

6-18 hours after fertilisation

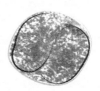

Day 2: cleaved embryo

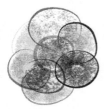

Day 3: 8 cell embryo

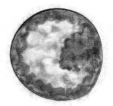

Day 5-6: blastocyst

Tocolytics

These are a group of drugs that were developed to try to reduce pre-term birth by stopping the uterus from contracting. Some fertility clinics may prescribe them before and after embryo transfer (ET) if you have experienced cramping for up to three days after ET on previous embryo transfers.

Total Testosterone Test

A man's testosterone levels will be checked during investigations into infertility. Testosterone is mainly produced by cells in his testes/testicles and also by the adrenal glands. Your ovaries also produce small amounts of testosterone and you may also have your levels checked during infertility investigations. See 'Testosterone' for more information.

Testosterone travels in your blood in two ways:

1. Attached to albumin proteins (one third) and sex hormone binding globulin or SHBG (two-thirds)

2. About 4% is free where it is not attached to any proteins.

A total testosterone test measures both free and attached testosterone, providing a more detailed picture of the testosterone levels in both your blood.

Traditional Chinese Medicine – TCM

Has been used for more than 2,500 years to prevent, diagnose and treat diseases, and includes acupuncture, herbal medicine, massage, diet, meditation and physical exercise.

It is based on the belief that your body's vital energy ('chi' or 'qi') circulates along channels ('meridians') that have branches connected to bodily organs and functions, and these keep your spiritual, emotional, mental and physical health in balance. It aims to restore your body's balance and harmony between the natural opposing forces of 'yin' and 'yang', which can block your 'chi' and cause disease. TCM is not a quick-fix treatment as you will need to commit to a treatment plan that covers months not weeks, and initially the treatments will be close together and will then gradually be less regular.

Where your fertility is concerned, TCM sees your reproductive system as a network of energy systems with each system being connected to organs and hormonal responses. This network is affected by stress, chemicals, poor diet, lack of exercise and excess emotions – all of which can put your body out of balance. For example, two of the most common organs in your body that are concerned with fertility are your liver and lungs, according to TCM. The liver is related to anger, stress, frustration, and desire and one of the most common TCM diagnoses for infertility is liver chi stagnation. The lungs are related to grief, sadness and holding on. In order to get your fertility 'chi' flowing you could use TCM to calm your mind through acupuncture, yoga or meditation.

A TCM practitioner will make a detailed assessment of your menstrual cycle, especially changes in the length of your cycles and menstrual bleeding to identify what, if any, changes are needed.

TCM may also help with male infertility, especially with improving a man's sperm count.

Like with a number of things concerned with infertility, there are doctors who support using TCM along with the more technical side of fertility treatments, such as IVF etc, and there are those who don't believe TCM has a place in Western medicine. Those doctors who don't have this belief is often because the theory and practice of TCM are not based upon scientific knowledge and there are not large studies to back up findings. However, some fertility clinics work closely with TCM practitioners, and they may even have an acupuncturist based at their clinic as there is a belief (though this is not proven), that having acupuncture just before and straight after embryo transfer (ET) can make a difference as to the embryo implanting successfully or not.

Always seek the advice of a certified TCM practitioner, do your research and, if you are wanting to combine TCM with fertility treatment, it is really important that you discuss this with your doctor.

> **Sheila says: You have no doubt read stories in magazines, newspapers and on the internet where women have been told they will never get pregnant or should use a donor egg, and they have tried TCM and have got pregnant naturally. I believe this is one of those treatments where you make up your own mind. After we did an IUI cycle that failed and then our first IVF cycle that also failed, I had several months of acupuncture and at the same time took herbal medicines, which did change my periods for the better so far as I was concerned. I didn't get pregnant naturally but my periods never went back to how they were before – which was a blessing in itself.**

Traditional Surrogacy

Also called 'straight', 'partial' and 'genetic surrogacy', this is when the surrogate becomes pregnant with her eggs and your partner's (or a donor's) sperm. The procedure is via intravaginal insemination (or artificial insemination as it used to be known as) either at home or at a clinic.

Because the surrogate's egg was used to get her pregnant, she will be the baby's biological mother, and therefore in the eyes of the law, she must give up her parental rights once the baby is born. This often makes it harder emotionally for both the surrogate and the intended parents (IPs) and is now less common than gestational surrogacy, (egg and sperm are from the IPs or donors).

However, it may be considered by the following because they will need to use a donor's egg anyway, so by using a traditional surrogate, the surrogate doubles as the egg donor:

- single men

- same-sex male couples
- intended mothers who cannot produce their own eggs.

Traditional surrogacy is much more complex from the legal aspect because the surrogate is the biological mother of the baby that is born. Also, the surrogate could change her mind about giving up the baby once the baby is born. It is very important that you seek legal advice in your own country regarding surrogacy laws as well as the laws in the surrogate's country, if she lives in a different country to you.

Transvaginal Ultrasound Scan – TVUS

This is a procedure where an ultrasound probe, often referred to as a 'wand', is placed into your vagina in order to see your womb, Fallopian tubes, ovaries, cervix and pelvic area. An ultrasound uses sound waves to obtain images and it gives higher quality images than if an abdominal ultrasound scan was performed.

You may have this scan if you are having investigations for infertility for the following reasons:

- unexplained vaginal bleeding
- painful periods
- to see if you have fibroids, cysts or uterine polyps.

During infertility treatment, such as IVF, you will have a number of scans to:

- evaluate and monitor how your follicles are developing
- monitor how your womb lining (endometrium) is thickening
- monitor ovulation

- during egg collection/retrieval.

Having a scan causes most of us some embarrassment (as do most fertility investigations!), may be uncomfortable (often due to the embarrassment), but shouldn't be painful.

The below is not to scale and is purely an artistic impression of your reproductive system.

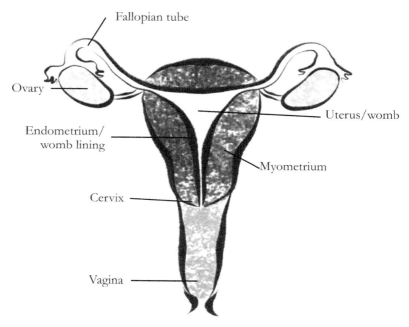

Triclosan

This is an antibacterial agent found in everyday household products such as soap, shampoo and toothpaste. It is known as an 'endocrine disrupter', meaning it interferes with naturally occurring hormones such as oestrogen/estrogen. It can affect sperm motility and the ability of the sperm to penetrate an egg, especially when a man is exposed to other harmful chemicals.

Trigger Shot

Once your fertility clinic has decided that your follicles are the correct size and your endometrium (womb lining) is a good thickness, you will be told when your egg collection/retrieval, EC/ER, will take place. In order to start the final maturation and release of the eggs, you will do an hCG (human chorionic gonadotropin) injection that mimics the luteinising hormone (LH) surge that brings about ovulation in a natural menstrual cycle.

This injection is known as the 'trigger shot' and it is usually done late in the evening roughly 36 hours before your egg collection/retrieval. Don't worry that you will ovulate before your egg collection/retrieval because natural ovulation wouldn't occur for 42-48 hours from the time of your injection. But the timing of this injection is very important for this very reason.

You may experience some discomfort after your trigger shot and, if you do, this is due to the ovaries being bigger than normal because of the stimulating drugs you have been taking.

Two-week Wait – TWW/2WW

This is a non-medical phrase that is greeted with both fear and excitement – rather like egg collection/retrieval and waiting to find out how many of your eggs have fertilised and are developing into lovely embryos.

It is the two weeks of time between having your embryo back safely inside your womb, and doing a pregnancy test that will give you an accurate result as to whether your fertility treatment has been successful or not. Doesn't sound too bad does it? For most of us, this is a rollercoaster on top of a rollercoaster on top of another rollercoaster emotional ride.

Usually you feel excited and positive in the first week and then, when the second week sets in, you start thinking 'this hasn't worked' and become anxious and stressed whilst being aware of every little spasm, ache and pain. You worry if they are early pregnancy symptoms or not.

You may have read loads of articles, blogs, forum posts etc on how to deal with the TWW; should you go back to work or not, is there anything you can eat to help implantation, can you exercise, how can you get through the two weeks without going insane, should you test early? So many questions and no one has the definitive answer.

If this is your first two-week wait you have no idea how you will feel during this time, and if it is your second, or third or more, you will probably agree that you have felt different during each one and maybe done things differently each time. This is understandable because if it didn't work the first time, you want to do something different the next time so that it works. One very important thing to remember is, if you do not get a positive pregnancy test or BFP, it is not because of something you did or didn't do during your TWW (providing you took the medical advice of your fertility clinic).

It can feel strange and lonely in this two-week period because the last few weeks have been all about scans, blood tests, appointments, injections, focusing on your follicles and womb lining, and then how many eggs have fertilised and have gone on to develop into embryos or blastocysts, and now you've nowhere to go and nothing to do but play a waiting game.

Remember everyone is different and everyone handles this time differently. Be gentle and kind to yourself and do what your gut instinct is telling you. By all means go on forums if that's your thing. If you have some cycle buddies (women who are going through their TWW the same time as you) they can be supportive but, remember, they are also going through their TWW and may not be coping so well, so if you need to excuse yourself because of things they are saying, that is fine. It is your TWW too. If you really don't want to go to work and can take the time off, do that and don't let anyone else tell you that you should be at work. If your work is very strenuous you may be able to get signed off anyway. If you want to spend your time visualising your embryo snuggling in and starting to grow, taking gentle walks, catching up on box sets or TV series or having a short break away from home, then do all these things if it helps the time to go by in the least stressful way.

The advice your clinic will give you will be more medical than emotional, though you may decide to see a counsellor or fertility coach during this time. Your clinic's advice will be along the lines of:

- do not lift anything heavy

- do not have hot baths or use a hot tub or visit a sauna/ steam room

- avoid rigorous exercise but gentle exercise, like walking, is fine

- keep taking any medication you have been prescribed – this is ensuring your hormones and womb lining are keeping your embryo safe and sound

- drink plenty of water to keep your womb lining nice and wet

- don't have sex even if you feel like it (that's probably due to the hormones); your womb has enough to do so don't overload it

- eat a healthy, balanced diet as this is far more important than eating just the foods that are supposed to aid implantation

- don't lie in bed as there is no evidence to show this helps with implantation

- spotting and bleeding is normal and doesn't necessarily mean this cycle hasn't worked; similarly, if you don't have any spotting this doesn't mean that your embryo hasn't implanted

- twinges and cramps are common and are nothing to worry about

- don't test early, hard though it is to stop yourself. If you test too early you may get a false positive or an incorrect negative result. You have had a lot of hormones in your body and are still taking hormones so this is why you could get an incorrect result. This is the reason why your clinic says don't test until test day; it's not because they are being mean.

Remember that your clinic and anyone you have told is rooting for you and wants you to get your BFP (positive pregnancy test) as much as you do. Good luck.

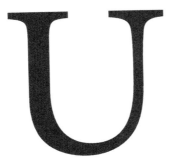

ULTRASOUND SCAN

to

UTERUS

It is estimated that over six million children have been conceived by IVF. (2016)

Ultrasound Scan – US, U/S

Sometimes called a 'sonogram', this is a procedure that uses high-frequency sound waves to create an image of a soft tissue structure inside your body, such as your womb or ovaries. A small device called a 'probe' or 'wand' is what gives off the high-frequency sound waves, but you can't hear them. When these sound waves bounce off your ovaries, for example, they create 'echoes' that are picked up by the probe and turned into a moving image that is displayed on a monitor whilst the scan is being carried out.

If you are having investigations into infertility or you are having fertility treatment, you will very likely have a lot of scans and these are usually internal scans rather than ones where the probe is moved over your abdomen. See 'Transvaginal Ultrasound Scan' for more information.

The below is not to scale and is purely an artistic impression of your reproductive system.

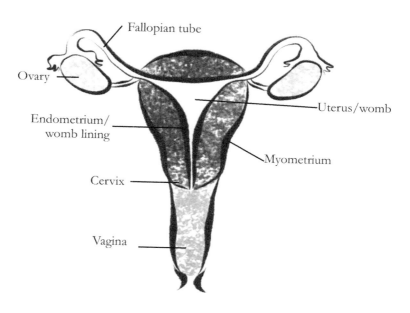

Fallopian tube

Ovary

Endometrium/
womb lining

Uterus/womb

Myometrium

Cervix

Vagina

Underweight

We usually think that it's only overweight women who are going to find it challenging to get pregnant, but if you are underweight you may find it takes longer to get pregnant too. Like being overweight, not every underweight woman is going to struggle – if you have a low body mass index (BMI), have a healthy diet and you don't obsessively exercise, it simply means that you are naturally thin and having fertility problems because you are underweight is quite unlikely. To find out more about your BMI see 'Body Mass Index' for more information. As a rough guide, if your BMI is under about 19 (the exact figure varies from country to country), you are considered to be 'underweight'.

If being underweight causes your hormones to be unbalanced this could affect ovulation and consequently your chances of getting pregnant. Compared to a woman who is a healthy weight, if you are underweight (not a healthy underweight as described above), you are more than twice as likely to take more than a year to get pregnant.

Being underweight affects your ovulation due to lack of body fat and, as body fat is where the body stores and uses oestrogen/ estrogen, this means you may not have enough oestrogen/ estrogen levels to support a normal menstrual cycle and so affects you ovulating. If you are underweight due to extreme exercising, so have low levels of body fat, your levels of oestradiol will be significantly lower which may lead to anovulation (you won't ovulate at all). The good news is that if you change your exercise habits and do less exercise and eat healthily, there is no reason why you shouldn't start to ovulate once your hormones are correctly balanced again.

However, if you are in the category where your exercise levels are normal and you eat healthily but you struggle to gain weight, you may want to consider the following:

1. Keep a detailed food diary of everything you eat for at least three days – record the number of calories you eat and how much protein, carbohydrates and fats you eat. This is often a surprising exercise (excuse the pun) because it may show you that you are not eating healthily for your fertility. Your goal is initially to put on 1-2lbs/453-907gms a week.

2. Eat five meals a day; either three meals with two or three snacks, or five small meals a day. This will make sure that you are getting the correct number of calories a day, and also that your blood sugar levels are consistent, which is essential for balanced hormone levels.

3. Plan your meals for a week or at least start with a day at a time. You need 2,200 calories a day so divide this between your meals and snacks every day.

4. Eat organic, whole fat, dairy, butter and yoghurt (organic so that you aren't eating/drinking excess hormones). If you have PCOS or endometriosis, it's better if you avoid dairy and have almond or coconut milk instead.

5. Eat foods that are dense in nutrients – this means that the level of the foods nutrients is high in relation to the number of calories that food contains. The nutrients you need to think about are vitamins, minerals, phytonutrients (found in plants), essential fatty acids and fibre.

Undescended Testicles

If your partner's testicles haven't descended (a condition called cryptorchidism) this can cause fertility issues because sperm and the male hormone testosterone are produced in his testicles. This isn't common nowadays as the operation to correct undescended testicles is carried out between five and fifteen months of age.

During pregnancy, a baby boy's testicles form inside his abdomen and they move down into the scrotum about a month or two before birth. However, it is not uncommon to find that in some baby boys one testicle doesn't descend. In rarer cases, both don't descend.

It is usually found out during the check-up just after birth and most will descend within the first three to six months of birth.

Unexplained Infertility – UI

This is when, despite you (and your partner) having routine fertility tests, no cause can be found as to why you are having problems getting pregnant. It may also be referred to as 'idiopathic infertility' and it affects about one in five couples.

It is an extremely difficult and frustrating diagnosis to accept because you know there has to be a reason. If you have a reason it is slightly more bearable because you know what you are dealing with and you can make informed choices, but when no one knows why, it is maddening. Some suggest that with further investigations and tests, and not just the basic ones, fewer people would be given this diagnosis. It is also quite likely that the cause hasn't been uncovered by science yet.

The diagnosis of unexplained increases as you age because you are more likely to have egg quantity and quality problems, but as there is no recognised fertility term for this, you are given the diagnosis of 'unexplained'.

It is suggested that if you are diagnosed with unexplained infertility of less than two years' duration, you have a good chance of getting pregnant over the next two years without using fertility treatment.

Possible causes of unexplained infertility are:

- anatomical abnormalities, such as the cilia (small hair-like structure) in your Fallopian tubes not moving the egg from your ovary to your womb, or there being scar tissue in your womb lining or Fallopian tubes; carrying out a vaginal ultrasound scan or hysteroscopy aids diagnosis better than just a laparoscopy

- abnormal development of the follicle and ovulation where an immature egg is released from the follicle rather than a mature egg, or the egg isn't released at all

- deformed egg structure or chromosome abnormalities in the egg

- luteal phase defect/abnormality, is where the number of days in your menstrual cycle after ovulation are too many or too less, so implantation is affected; investigations can include examining samples from your womb lining (endometrial biopsy) or monitoring, by blood tests, the levels of the hormones progesterone and prolactin on different days after ovulation.

If you are not satisfied with a diagnosis of unexplained infertility you may find it beneficial to get a second opinion – a new pair of eyes looking at your results may bring something to light that has been missed, or a different specialist may have different ideas. Not knowing the cause of your infertility means that anything is possible and you are only limited by your own ability to think outside of the box and current available resources.

When you have this diagnosis, it is very difficult to know when to decide that 'enough is enough' because you are so hopeful that, when you have another test done and another investigation carried out, the cause will be found out. It is very hard to move on and either grieve or make plans for a life without children. It may be worth speaking to a fertility counsellor if you find yourself stuck and unable to make decisions about your future.

> **Sheila says: We were given a diagnosis of 'unexplained' and for us, we didn't agree because there is always an explanation of some kind. The way I see it is that fertility is not simple because there is so much involved – hormones, eggs, womb, womb lining – not forgetting that there are two people who need to make a baby, so what's going on with the sperm also has to be factored in. With most other medical conditions like diabetes, cardiovascular issues and high blood pressure, the causes are more recognisable so easier to treat, and it is just that one person who has it.**

Unicornuate Uterus

This is a congenital (meaning you were born with it) abnormality of your uterus and it occurs when the Müllerian ducts form your uterus, Fallopian tubes and ovaries. Your uterus is usually half the size of one without this abnormality and has what is called a 'rudimentary horn' on one side, which may or may not be connected to your uterus. It is not uncommon that you only have one Fallopian tube. You usually wouldn't know you had a unicornuate uterus until you have investigations into why you can't get pregnant and have had recurrent miscarriages. Approximately 2-8% of women who have investigations into infertility have this type of uterus.

Diagnosis is made by having a hysterosalpingogram or ultrasound; for more information go to these terms in this book. Currently there is no surgical treatment for this condition but some women have the rudimentary horn removed, as this can cause serious complications if an embryo does implant there rather than in the uterus itself.

Should you get pregnant, there is a very high risk that the pregnancy will end in an early miscarriage or rupture of the horn if that is where the embryo has implanted. However, there are women who have safely delivered their baby when they have a unicornuate uterus as no two women will have exactly the same abnormality. The advice given is that, if you can cope psychologically with experiencing recurrent miscarriages, keep trying, and when you do get pregnant and the pregnancy is developing beyond a few weeks, ensure that you are very carefully monitored and be prepared that you may have a premature baby. There was a woman with a unicornuate uterus who had 17 miscarriages before she had a baby and another woman had twins.

Urologist

This is a trained doctor who has specialised in the study or treatment of the functionality and disorders of the male and female urinary system, and the male reproductive system.

You may be referred to a urologist if you need treatment for a condition concerned with any of the following:

- bladder, such as incontinence, prolapse
- urethra, such as urinary tract infection (UTI)
- ureters
- kidneys, such as kidney failure, transplant, stones
- adrenal glands

A man may be referred if he has fertility issues such as:

- varicocele
- retrograde ejaculation
- sperm antibodies
- blockage in the testicles.

Uterine Lining

The medical term is endometrium. See this term for more information.

Uterus

Also called your womb. This is part of your reproductive tract and its main function is to carry your baby until s/he is born. It weighs about 60 grams, is shaped like an upside-down pear and is in the middle of your pelvis, behind your bladder and in front of your rectum. The position of the uterus can be:

- anteverted, where it tips slightly forwards
- retroverted, where is bends slightly backwards.

There are four parts to the uterus:

1. Fundus – this is the upper part of the uterus and the Fallopian tubes attach to the uterus just below it

2. Corpus – this is the main part of the uterus and stretches with your growing baby. The lining is the endometrium and it is this that changes in its thickness during your menstrual cycle. When a fertilised egg arrives in the uterus it attaches to the endometrium and if a fertilised egg doesn't attach, the endometrium is shed during menstruation. See 'Endometrium' for more information.

3. Isthmus – this is the part of the uterus where it narrows between the corpus and the cervix

4. Cervix – this is the lowest part of the uterus and connects to the vagina. Glands in the lining of the cervix usually

produce a thick cervical mucus, but around the time of ovulation it becomes thinner, enabling sperm to swim more easily into the uterus.

Some conditions of the uterus that may make it more difficult for you to get pregnant are:

- endometriosis
- fibroids
- pelvic inflammatory disease (PID).

For more information on these conditions – see the relevant term in this book.

There are also abnormalities of the uterus that you may be born with (congenital) that can also affect your chances of getting pregnant, namely a septate uterus or a unicornuate uterus. For more information on these conditions – see the relevant term in this book.

The symptoms of many uterine conditions are the same and these are the common ones:

- very heavy periods
- bleeding between periods
- pelvic or lower-back pain
- pain during menstruation or sex
- nasty smelling vaginal discharge
- pain when you wee and poo.

Conditions in the uterus need to be perfect in order that an embryo implants successfully and stays there for nine months.

The below is not to scale and is purely an artistic impression of your reproductive system.

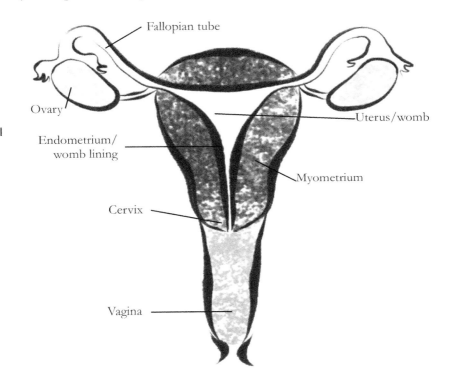

V & W

VAGINAL ULTRASOUND

to

WATER

In 2016, there were 82,000 IVF cycles in the UK. 20,340 of these resulted in a live birth and 61,660 didn't. (HFEA)

Vaginal Steaming

Also known as 'V-Steaming' and 'yoni steaming' ('yoni' being the Sanskrit word for womb or vagina – or bajos from Mayan healers). It is an ancient herbal treatment that is used by healers to cleanse and revitalise your womb, effectively reducing menstrual discomfort. It may also be used to:

- reduce discomfort, bloating and exhaustion associated with your menstrual cycle
- decrease a heavy menstrual flow as well as brown/dark/purple blood
- regulate irregular or absent menstrual cycles
- treat uterine fibroids and ovarian cysts
- help with infertility, especially when used with abdominal massage.

The healers who use it believe the herbal steam:

- increases circulation
- thins the mucus
- cleanses the whole reproductive system.

As with most things to do with fertility, some will say vaginal steaming doesn't do anything and others will swear by it. If you want to try it, I would strongly suggest that you find a practitioner who can help and advise you and do not consider it without seeking professional advice if you are currently doing fertility treatment.

Vaginal Ultrasound

See 'Transvaginal Ultrasound Scan' for more information.

Varicocele

A varicocele is an enlargement of the veins inside the scrotum which contains the testicles; imagine them like a varicose vein in the leg. Often there are no signs or symptoms that a man has a varicocele until he is having investigations into infertility, because a varicocele can cause a low sperm count and poor sperm quality. If there is pain and/or noticeable swelling he should seek medical help immediately. Over time varicoceles may become more enlarged and visible and can cause a swollen testicle, usually on the left side.

Why varicoceles occur is not known but it is thought they form when the valves inside the veins in the spermatic cord (which carries blood to and from the testicles) prevent blood from flowing properly, resulting in the veins widening or dilating.

The reason why a varicocele may cause infertility is due to damage to sperm production and function from the excess heat caused by the blood pooling, and oxidative stress (ROS) on sperm.

Repair of a varicocele is done to improve fertility and it is either a surgical or non-surgical procedure:

Surgical procedure – can be done as an outpatient under local or general anaesthetic. A small cut is made in the abdomen close to where the testicles originally descended (testicles originally form in the abdomen when a baby boy is in the womb). The veins that produce the varicocele are cut to stop further blood flow to the varicocele.

Non-surgical procedure – called 'percutaneous embolisation', this repairs the varicocele and is done under a local anaesthetic. A small catheter is inserted through a large vein in the groin or neck and passed until it reaches the varicocele, where it is blocked off by a balloon, a coil or medication.

Some experts believe having surgery will improve sperm production and quality whereas others believe the surgery makes no difference and until larger studies are carried out, it is advisable that you ask questions of your doctor and/or seek a second opinion, if you feel it will help you to make a decision.

Vitamin B6

It is very common these days to find that you are deficient in Vitamin B6 – deficiency can cause irregular menstrual cycles, imbalance of the hormone progesterone and poor egg and sperm development. Your levels of Vitamin B6 can be checked by having a blood test.

Vitamin B12

Having adequate levels of Vitamin B12 may help with the development of your endometrium (womb lining) and could therefore decrease the chance of having a miscarriage. Being deficient in this vitamin may lead to irregular ovulation and, if severe enough, ovulation may completely stop.

Deficiency in men may affect sperm quality and production.

Your levels of Vitamin B12 can be checked by having a blood test.

Vitamin D

This is a fat-soluble vitamin produced when you are exposed to the sun. Sitting in the sun for only 15-20 minutes a day will create between 10,000-25,000 IU (international units) of vitamin D. However, due to using sun screen to prevent skin cancer most of us have very low levels of vitamin D. It can also be absorbed by the body when you eat foods, mainly eggs, wild caught salmon, beef liver and dairy, and it is also added to some foodstuffs – you can see it on the packaging. Due to the fat-soluble nature of this vitamin, it is slow to be absorbed and, if you take a supplement, it can sometimes take six to twelve months before the levels in your blood are normal.

The level of vitamin D3 in your body can affect your chances of getting pregnant because it is needed by your body to make the sex hormones (oestrogen/estrogen and testosterone) – this is the case for you and for men. If you have sufficient levels of vitamin D3, you are almost twice as likely to conceive compared to women you have insufficient levels of vitamin D3. Where fertility treatment is concerned, it is believed that women who had good levels of vitamin D3 were more likely to produce good quality eggs and implantation of an embryo was more successful in women with adequate levels of vitamin D3.

Outside of fertility, vitamin D also plays a crucial role in:

- normal cell division
- normal functioning of the immune system
- strong teeth and bones (you may have heard of 'rickets', which is common in children who do not get enough vitamin D)
- preventing dementia
- reducing cancer risks
- treating depression naturally.

It is almost impossible to overdose on vitamin D and it is important for you to have adequate levels when you are trying to get pregnant as well as your partner, if you are using his sperm. A healthy level is 20 nonograms/millilitre to 50 ng/ml and a level less than 12 ng/ml indicates a deficiency. If you want to have a blood test, it is called '25-hydroxyvitamin D' or 25(OH)D.

Vitrification

See 'Egg Freezing' and/or 'Embryo Freezing' for more information.

Water

Drink at least eight 8 oz or 225ml glasses of pure water a day. Dehydration can cause many issues in your body but specific to fertility, it causes blood thickening and decreases blood circulation. Adequate water intake will flush out toxins from your body, ensure the quality and amount of cervical fluid is ideal for conception, prevent urine infections, and before and during the two-week wait, ensures your womb lining is wet and spongy. For men, drinking more water can help increase his ejaculate and improve sperm production.

X & Y

XENOHORMONES

to

YOGA

84% of women of childbearing age have cramps during their menstrual cycles. This is known as dysmenorrhea.

Xenohormones

These are man-made, toxic substances that are easily absorbed through your skin and by your body and build up over time. They have a hormonal effect on your body. The most frequently occurring xenohormones are xenoestrogens, which mimic the effects of oestrogen/estrogen and thus cause progesterone deficiency. They damage developing tissues in your endocrine system, which includes your thyroid, adrenal glands, pituitary gland, testicles, ovaries and the pancreas.

The extent of the damage to cells/tissues does depend on your age when you are exposed to xenohormones – so a developing baby's tissues will be very sensitive to any exposure and may cause irreparable damage that does not become apparent until the baby has grown up and is an adult.

For example, at about day 18-23 after conception, the baby's gonads are developing. If a baby boy is exposed to xenohormones, his Sertoli cells in the testicles maybe damaged, which could affect his sperm count when he is older. If a baby girl is exposed, her follicle cells in her ovaries maybe damaged and this can affect her ovaries and their ability to ovulate, or a lack of progesterone production, making her oestrogen/estrogen dominant and prone to having early miscarriages.

Xenohormones come from:

- solvents and adhesives, such as paint and varnish, nail polish, glue and cleaning products
- plastic food containers, drinking bottles, plastic food wraps
- personal care products, such as perfumes, skin cleansers, antiperspirants, sun screen

- non-organic livestock which are fed oestrogenic drugs to fatten them up
- pesticides, herbicides and fungicides that are sprayed on crops, on the lawn and weeds
- anything made from mineral oil, which is made from crude oil which also makes motor oil for cars – baby oil is made from 100% mineral oil
- emulsifiers found in soaps and make-up.

What you can do to minimise your exposure are the following:

- do not microwave food in plastic containers nor cover food when storing or microwaving with plastic food wrap
- do not leave plastic drinking bottles in the sun
- eat organic and locally grown and in-season foods as far as possible
- peel non-organic fruits and vegetables
- eat organic meat and dairy
- stop using pesticides etc and use organic products
- use natural skin care products and ones that don't contain mineral oil
- use natural feminine care products
- use unbleached paper products, such as toilet roll, kitchen towel
- use a water filter rather than buying bottled water
- avoid processed and packaged food.

Yoga

This can be beneficial if you are trying to get pregnant as it uses key poses that help to nurture, support and strengthen the endocrine and reproductive system. With the endocrine system being essential for hormonal balance, it is as important to use poses that promote healthy endocrine function as it is to use poses that support the whole reproductive system.

Yoga is also known to reduce stress, anxiety and depression and these are all common when dealing with fertility challenges.

Some of the benefits of fertility yoga are:

- helping to reset your endocrine system and so balance your hormones
- increases circulation to your reproductive system
- strengthens your abdomen and lower back
- opens your hip area in preparation for conception
- it may help to clear adhesions and blockages in your reproductive organs
- it supports a healthy immune system.

Some yoga poses are:

- Bhramari Pranayama – relieves stress, anxiety and worry
- Paschimottanasana – vitalises your ovaries and womb
- Supta Baddha Konasana – exercises your inner thigh and groin muscles, relieves menstrual cramps and other discomforts that come with fertility treatments
- Sarvangasana – stimulates your thyroid gland, calms your mind and relieves stress
- Bhujangasana – increases the blood flow to your ovaries and womb

- Setu Bandhasana – helps your pelvic region open up and expand and stimulates your thyroid.

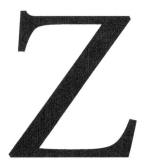

ZINC to
ZYGOTE INTRAFALLOPIAN
TRANSFER

An estimated 200 million women worldwide are affected by
endometriosis

Zinc

Having adequate levels of zinc is important in you and in men and a deficiency can cause chromosome changes causing infertility and an increase in the risk of having a miscarriage.

In you, it is necessary so that you can make use of the essential fertility hormones oestrogen/estrogen and progesterone.

In men, a large amount of zinc is found in sperm, and it is necessary to make the outer layer and tail of the sperm. A deficiency of zinc affects sperm count. Levels of zinc can be tested, so you may wish to look into this.

Zygote Intrafallopian Transfer – ZIFT

This was similar to IVF in that eggs were collected/retrieved after your ovaries had been stimulated and then your eggs and the sperm were allowed to fertilise. Once a fertilised egg has become two cells, usually within 24 hours, is it called a 'zygote' and it is the zygote that was transferred to your Fallopian tube using a laparoscopy. It is no longer carried out as IVF is more successful.

The below is not to scale and is purely an artistic impression of IVF.

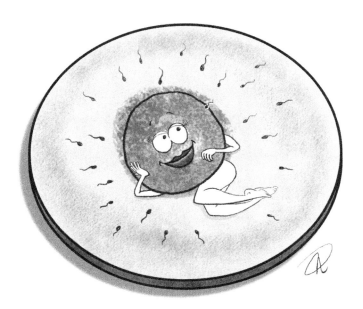

Thank you for purchasing this book and if you have found the information in this book interesting and helpful, please let others know that it is available so that they too can be helped on their journey. If you would like to leave a review, this also help others to make a decision.

You may not know about my free ebook 'The Best Fertility Jargon Buster: the most concise A-Z list of fertility abbreviations and acronyms you will ever need'. If you would like your own ebook copy, please go to this link: www.mfsbooks.co.uk

The Best Fertility Jargon Buster

Over 200 "fertility forum" abbreviations

The most concise A-Z list of fertility abbreviations and acronyms you will ever need.

SHEILA LAMB

Founder of My Fertility Specialist magazine

Thank you for reading

Sheila Lamb

Index

Printed in Great Britain
by Amazon